"This book is a roadmap to lifelong health based upon a natural, holistic and effective approach. From understanding the brain's physiology and the role your mindset plays in your overall health, to the extensive list of natural remedies and nutrient-rich foods, each chapter is packed with one breakthrough insight after another."

— Dr. Joe Rubino
founder of www.CenterForPersonalReinvention.com
Creator, www.TheSelfEsteemBook.com and
www.HighSelfEsteemKids.com

"Anyone interested in finding or regaining health must read this book. Filled with witty, valuable tips and strategies, *Turn Back the Clock* provides an easy-to-follow plan that emphasizes the importance of nourishing, supporting, and stimulating our brain, eating real food, using the appropriate supplements, and how to set and achieve goals. Dr. Crawford is an inspiration!"

— Keith Leon, speaker, book mentor & best-selling author of the book,
Who Do You Think You Are? Discover The Purpose Of Your Life

"Get inspired to make good choices and live more healthfully, vibrantly and youthfully with the tips and advice that Dennis K. Crawford offers in his new book *Turn Back the Clock*."

— Lisa Coffey, author of *What's Your Dosha, Baby?*
and founder of www.CoffeyTalk.com

"The information provided in this book can help people make necessary decisions, as they age gracefully, for the rest of their lives."

— Patricia Noel Drain CPC, CSP
Speaker, Author & Business Mentor, www.PatriciaDrain.com

D0921928

"*Turn Back the Clock* is a great piece of writing. The bottom line in life is our health is our responsibility, not something we can delegate to others. With his intelligence, concise writing style, and dry wit, Dennis cuts through the conflicting health information and aids us in taking action and creating our own anti-aging program. Dennis has a knack for taking complex subjects and breaking them down for easy consumption so we can make the best decisions. Health is not just the absence of disease but also incorporates our quality of life. Dennis brings information together in a holistic manner feeding our body, mind, and spirit. The concepts are simple and presented clearly, making *Turn Back the Clock* quick reading and the ideas easy to implement. I recommend *Turn Back the Clock* to all who wish to improve their life on any level while understanding and enjoying the process."

— Tamara Dorris, author of *Get Well Now*
and host of www.InLoveWithSacto.com

"Dr. Crawford's out-of-the-box thinking gives insights into managing our health in ways that aren't traditionally taught through allopathic treatment. I'm passionate about supporting our health in alternative ways and getting to the truth, so we can get to the root, rather than maintaining an unacceptable status quo of low energy, pain, being overweight, and I love that Dr. Crawford takes this on so powerfully, in his practice and in this book. *Turn Back the Clock* is choc full of tips and insights that will help you live a healthy, energetic, and happy life. Just by implementing a couple of the gems he reveals—you could change your life! His book is full of wisdom and secrets 'they' don't want us to know that will help you take responsibility for your own health and choices. He makes it easy for you to educate yourself and make better choices. Thanks, Dr. Crawford, for being a pioneer, doing your own research, taking a 'whole-istic' and realistic approach, and pushing the boundaries of Western medicine to share all you do."

— Louise Crooks, The Keys to Clarity!
Coach, Business Coach to Holistic Practitioners
Integrative Doctors & Coaches, www.keystoclarity.com

"Dr. Dennis K. Crawford is not only a fine physician of the processes of wellness, he attends to people, really attends to their particular wellness and promotes the balance required to live a fully self expressed life. I truly respect him and know that this book will be of service to those that let themselves be served by the years of applied knowledge and care to which Dr. Crawford has dedicated himself."

— Rev. Bruce Kellogg
Unity Minister, Cottonwood, AZ

"If you wish to develop your physical and mental health, this is the book for you. Dr. Crawford spells out the pathways for you to follow. Beginning with self-analysis to identify the areas that may need improvement, you can achieve your ambitions with the aid of this book. Good medicine does not always taste sweet and so it is with Dr. Crawford's advice. However, he speaks the truth which is derived from his knowledge obtained from his years of experience in the natural health field."

— Dr. Milne Ongley, MD

"Six months shy of my 30th birthday, I was diagnosed with idiopathic thrombocytopenia. This is a life threatening auto-immune disease where antigens attach to platelets in the blood, then the spleen destroys these platelets, causing a low platelet count. After several months of drug therapy with no results, my doctor wanted to remove my spleen. I was not comfortable with that approach. I began seeing Dr. Crawford who recommended a regimen of specific herbs, enzymes, and diet. My platelet count eventually normalized and remains normal years later. I am healthy, I still have my spleen, and I have Dr. Crawford to thank for it!"

— Allison Dampier
Director/Co-Founder Advantages Private School

"*Turn Back the Clock* is a great piece of writing. The bottom line in life is our health is our responsibility, not something we can delegate to others. With his intelligence, concise writing style, and dry wit, Dennis cuts through the conflicting health information and aids us in taking action and creating our own anti-aging program. Dennis has a knack for taking complex subjects and breaking them down for easy consumption so we can make the best decisions. Health is not just the absence of disease but also incorporates our quality of life. Dennis brings information together in a holistic manner feeding our body, mind, and spirit. The concepts are simple and presented clearly, making *Turn Back the Clock* quick reading and the ideas easy to implement. I recommend *Turn Back the Clock* to all who wish to improve their life on any level while understanding and enjoying the process."

— Christine Issel, M.A., National board certified reflexologist
and author of *Reflexology: Art, Science and History*
Reflexognosy: A Shift in Paradigm; and *Eunice Ingham: A Biography*

"*Turn Back the Clock* is full of very useful information that all of us desperately need in this world of stress and toxicity. If you or anyone you know wants to live a longer, healthier life, then this is the guide book. This book will appeal to the average person looking to improve his or her health, as well as the "anti-aging" expert, and everyone in between. I highly recommend it."

— Dr. Kathy Acquistapace, D.C. N.D.

"Dr. Crawford brilliantly brings fresh new research and information to those seeking a holistic, natural approach to lifelong health. He has a delightful way with words that makes this complete guide to naturally reprogramming your mind and body easy to understand and implement."

— Bessie Jo Tillman, MD

"Our family has been blessed by Dr. Crawford's training, abilities, and gifts for the past 13 years. It began when he found the cause of my wife's infertility. As a result, we have two wonderful children. Dr. Crawford then found and treated the cause of my knee pain, averting surgery. Again, when my wife and I begged pediatricians to find out why our daughter was so sick, Dr. Crawford figured out, in one visit, that she had a gluten allergy. He helped us heal her intestines, and we believe it saved her life. He has also treated our son for seasonal allergies, colds, and flues. Whatever the ailment, Dr. Crawford is the one we go to and whom we recommend to all our friends."

— John Cabigas, Major, USAF (Ret.), Former U-2 pilot

"A must read for anyone serious about embracing a natural approach to an improved life—at any age. Dr. Crawford's successful Clinical Herbal Applications applied in his practice clearly reveals personal, practical, and positive results experienced over many years in a myriad of individual cases!"

— Charlie W. Jordan, CMH, DOM
Certified Medical Herbalist, Doctor of Oriental Medicine

"My son Ross is autistic. Through a chain of events, we found Dr. Crawford. At this point we were exhausted, very scared and hopeless as Ross was worse than ever. When Dr. Crawford evaluated Ross and said, "I know that you are feeling bad now, but you will get better," I felt as though someone has just breathed life into me. I had hope for the first time in months. Dr. Crawford was honest and said the treatment would take time. We followed his instructions to the letter and now Ross is much more alert, communicative, healthy, fun, loves people, looks them straight in the eye, has become independent in his self-help skills, tells jokes, and continues to get well to this day."

— Linneal Weimar, proud mother

"I first started seeing Dr. Crawford over 25 years ago. Since then I have never needed the services of traditional allopathic medicine. I am happy to recommend Dr. Crawford to you. The strategies outlined in this book are a 'must-know' for those who want to stop worrying about the future. In simple language, he lays out specific, proven steps to create cutting edge results —now. I am living proof."

— Sean West, Las Vegas Musician and Nightclub Owner

"Great read. Very informative. Full of all the wonderful information you grow to expect from Dr. Crawford. He has an incredible amount of knowledge and is truly a great educator. I highly recommend this book for anyone interested in having a healthy, happy life."

— Sandy Smith, Medical Assistant, Nutritional Consultant

Turn Back the Clock

Seven Steps to More Youthful Living

Turn
Back
the Clock

Seven Steps to More Youthful Living

by
Dr. Dennis K. Crawford

First Edition
10 9 8 7 6 5 4 3 2

Book Cover design by Cathi Stevenson
www.bookcoverexpress.com

Book Edited by Heather Marsh
www.classicediting.com

Interior Design by Rudy Milanovich and Keith Leon

ISBN: 978-1466314504

Dr. Dennis K. Crawford
Fair Oaks, CA
www.crawfordnaturalhealthcenter.com

Contents

Acknowledgements 13

Introduction 15

chapter ONE: You are as Young as Your Brain Allows 19

chapter TWO: Energy Is Everything 41

chapter THREE: Stop Worrying, Start Living 63

chapter FOUR: Watch Out for Gopher Holes 85

chapter FIVE: Nature's Pharmacy 105

chapter SIX: Beyond Food 141

chapter SEVEN: The Turn Back the Clock Mindset 163

Conclusion 189

Index 191

ACKNOWLEDGEMENTS

I would like to thank the following people:

Keith Leon: You got my attention with your incredible singing. To find out you were also a best-selling author and a coach to other aspiring authors wanting to get their book ideas into print was icing on the cake. Your friendship, support, and expertise are appreciated more than I can express. You were truly the right person at the right time to come into my life. Thank you.

Heather Marsh: Your attention to the details is very much appreciated. What you do goes far beyond that, however. I always felt I was talking to a caring, supportive friend or therapist. Your patience, kindness, and always being there means a lot to me. By helping people like myself to get information out there, you are making a big difference. Thank you for being on my team.

My Patients: I am honored and grateful that you have entrusted me as a partner to help you achieve your health goals. Working with you is a privilege I don't take lightly. I can assist, coach, and make suggestions but I know that when you decide upon a natural approach, it requires taking personal responsibility. That is why many people haven't chosen this path, but you have. I greatly appreciate your proactivity. I am fortunate to have the opportunity to work with such wonderful people on a daily basis. While I don't always hit home runs, I am always learning from you, my teachers. Often "failures" led to knowledge that helped many of my subsequent patients.

Thank you to all my friends who have supported me with this book and for your continued words of encouragement, not only with this project, but in everyday life as well. It means a lot to know you are always there.

My mother: Thank you for all your love and support. While I have not always been the ideal son, you always believed in me. You saw the good in me when I (and many others) couldn't see it. Whenever I achieved a milestone like graduating from college you would say, "I always knew you could do it." Knowing I always had you cheering for me has been such a blessing and has helped me get through the really tough times. I love you and I can't thank you enough for your faith in me.

INTRODUCTION

I didn't think the screams would ever stop. They were shrill, intense, and continuous. As a parent, I intuitively gauged the severity of his cries. Before this day, most were nothing to worry about, but these cries were different. They were unfamiliar sounds powered by too much pain.

The day before my son seemed so perfect: Darren was six months old, happy, fun, and full of life. Today things were different. A "routine" checkup at the pediatrician's office resulted in a "routine" vaccine given. There was no warning about possible side effects. Call after call to the doctor proved futile, but eventually I got a nurse on the phone. She assured me this was a "normal" reaction with some children. "Nothing to worry about." I was a typical, uneducated parent who trusted the information doctors gave me. Of course, I wanted to believe her, but I knew there was nothing "normal" about the pain my son was experiencing. He was not the same after that September day and, in the weeks that followed, his health deteriorated rapidly.

That day marked a dramatic change in my life, too. I began a deliberate search for medical treatment to reclaim my son's health. I did not set out to become a doctor. I was just looking for answers that didn't come. Endless doctor's visits led to a growing list of medications to treat his symptoms. As serious side effects of drugs started to surface, including his passing blood, the medical response was always the same: more drugs for the symptoms. Yet no doctor could tell me why his physical health was poor, nor was any advice given to regain it. It was a vicious cycle.

When I really saw the futility of this path, I decided to do something different. I didn't feel I had any choice. The one major problem, however, was I didn't have the slightest idea what to do next. I knew that drugs could save lives and we had an excellent medical system when it came to treating trauma and disease, but restoring health in the absence of these two elements was a different issue. None of the well-meaning doctors whom we met even addressed that. Every approach focused on relieving short-term symptoms.

Eventually, I started a trial and error system of exploration. We started seeing chiropractors, nutritionists, acupuncturists, energetic healers, and everything in between. While there were clearly benefits to many of these visits, I still felt something was missing. Many in the natural field still focused on symptoms, or they were limited by their expertise in a particular technique. I found I would have to put this whole picture together on my own.

I began reading health books and taking courses while still searching for doctors that might help. I remember thinking, "It shouldn't be this difficult to learn how to get well." During this process, I was exposed to a new world that I became keenly interested in. The philosophy of natural medicine seemed rational to me: The body heals itself. If the body can't heal itself, there is something blocking the healing, or it doesn't have the resources to heal. I saw the universal law of cause and effect applied to health as much as anything else in our lives. Each book I read or class I took always led to another, and eventually I became a Doctor of Chiropractic, with certifications in Botanical Medicine and Enzyme Therapeutics.

I have been asked many times over the years to write a book. My first recollection was about 25 years ago when a well-known psychic, whom I had not previously met, came in as a patient and her first words to me were, "Start writing your book." I actually did start a few times over the years, but never completed it. I did not yet feel I was contributing much that had not already been said in other books. I wanted to give readers a unique perspective on wellness. I now feel I have accomplished that.

This book is about possibilities and empowerment. It is designed to provide self-motivated people with an overview of the various ingredients necessary to be healthy and productive at any age. The most common blocks to healing are covered, as well as an extensive list of proven natural remedies. It is not a one-size-fits-all health book. People are more complex than that. You could be eating healthy, for example, but if you can't digest your food (Chapter 4), or your brain isn't working optimally (Chapter 1), or you are in a constant state of fear and worry (Chapter 3), you are not going to reap the benefits of your healthy efforts.

This book is meant to provide many of the answers I wished I had when I was desperately looking for them. I desire to provide that service to those currently in the same situation I faced.

My son is doing well today. The doctors who treated his whole body, and determined the right therapy at the right time, got him back on a path to improved health. That is the model I still adhere to in my practice.

To the many who have asked me to write a book over the years, alas, here it is. Thank you for your patience. I hope this becomes the right book at the right time for you.

Dr. Dennis K. Crawford

chapter ONE

YOU ARE AS YOUNG AS YOUR BRAIN ALLOWS

Inside your body, your brain runs the show. It conducts the symphony. Most health and personal development information often ignores the brain. The body gets a lot of attention, so does behavior. Both require a healthy functioning brain.

Life is as simple as this: Your level of vitality and wellness is directly related to how healthy your brain is. When the brain thrives, you thrive.

Of course, the reverse is also true. When your brain is not nourished or supported, the rest of your body can't thrive. If it is fed a constant diet of fake food, routine activities, and uninspired thinking, the results are undesirable.

Many people live like this. They find a comfort zone that gets them by in the world and then stay where it feels safe. They eat the same ten foods every day, watch the same television shows, think the same thoughts, and so on. After all, living this way has gotten them this far, so it must be working. Right?

Absolutely not true.

What is wrong with living habitually? Nothing, if your ambition is to just exist until you die. This approach to life is also a death sentence to the brain. The longer you live this way, the more dead your brain becomes. After awhile, you can't even conceive of the possibility that you are not alive, in the sense that you are not living a life. You are living a lie. The lie is that you think you are fully awake, yet, if you are like most people, you are actually sleepwalking.

To wake up from this nightmare and turn back the clock, two things must happen. The first key is being open to the possibility that there are areas in life where you are not 100% present. This is the beginning of an awakening process which will start opening the doors to your true potential. This self-examination is not always easy or pleasant, which is why most people prefer not do it.

How interesting it is that existing without self-examination also creates resistance. Instead of jumping at the chance to change, people will often do the opposite. They will resist change and make excuses to justify selling themselves out to mediocrity and less. They will even become resistant to change within themselves. It is an amazing phenomenon to observe. Stagnation, boredom, depression, dullness, inflexibility, aches, and pains are all too common consequences of this living hell.

The second key to improving your quality of life and turning back the clock is to ensure that your brain and body have the resources to function optimally. The brain is no different from any other part of the body in that it needs certain essential ingredients to thrive. It is a live, dynamic organ, the most metabolically active in the whole body. It is important to do the right things, in the right order, to get lasting results. To not give the brain top priority is to put the cart before the horse.

I will discuss these two keys, along with proven strategies that will feed, stimulate, and revive your marvelous brain. I will also explore another major player regarding optimal brain function: the degree of inflammation a person has. Inflammation in the brain can literally burn it out, with dementia as a possible result.

I will elaborate more on these essential brain needs later, but since it is so important to everything else regarding our health and behavior, does it not seem logical that the brain should be our major concern in our effort to turn back our biological clock?

To start with, it is necessary to understand that an adequate oxygen supply to the brain is of paramount importance. To do so requires a healthy heart and circulatory system, healthy blood, and regular exercise. Most approaches that benefit the heart and circulation, will also promote increased blood flow and oxygen availability to the brain. 20% of all our oxygen is used by the brain, so it only makes sense that anything which increases oxygen utilization by the brain is a good thing. Of course, the reverse is also true. Anything that decreases oxygen supply to the brain is harmful.

Circulation to the brain is crucial, so obviously a healthy heart and circulatory system are essential. The brain also requires a steady supply of glucose. One's life and moods can be a reflection of the glucose availability to the brain. Erratic blood sugar can lead to an erratic life filled with many emotional highs and lows, memory problems, and a general lack of control over one's life.

When blood sugar is out of balance, it will usually spike too high after a meal, particularly after the person eats carbo-hydrates. At this time, a person may feel abnormally high or happy, but that feeling will be temporary because when the blood sugar is brought down, it goes too far down. The tendency when this happens is to become emotionally low, have short-term memory loss, headaches, dizziness or even fainting, and there could be strong cravings for sugar or alcohol to bring the blood sugar back up. This yo-yo of highs and lows can make people feel like they are losing their minds. It has ended many marriages and has been part of the reason why some people have made poor choices and, in extreme cases, have even ended up in prison.

Exercise, for all of its fitness attributes, is not an option, it is mandatory. When you exercise, the body actually makes more mitochondria in the cells. This is where energy is made. So, more energy-producing powerhouses are produced and you begin an upward trend of producing more energy, having more energy, and feeling like exercising more, which produces more energy. A lack of exercise is a very common cause of depleted energy. I realize a lot of people are too tired to exercise, but as they get more rest they can ease into an exercise program.

What a great vicious cycle this is! Besides the increased energy, other benefits of exercise are an increase in decision-making reaction time, improved self-esteem and moods, a decrease in stress, a slowing of the aging process and better sleep. You build momentum that makes you unstoppable.

It is not necessary to run marathons for exercise. In fact, it is best if you do not. Easy, prolonged exercise that you enjoy doing is best. Cycling or using any of the many types of cardio fitness machines available is fine. Find what you like and stick to it. Exercising consistently is the key. Obviously, if you have a specific training goal, like to increase muscle mass or do a triathlon, you would need to tailor your exercise routine to accomplish that objective. For the average person who is looking to get fit, perhaps lose a few pounds, and increase their level of wellness, the main goal is to find something enjoyable and do it regularly.

Do not over exert yourself or engage in any exercise that causes pain or aggravates an old injury. It should feel good to do, not painful. The idea is to increase circulation, and get fit mentally and physically. Overexertion is stress, and requires sugar burning for fuel. The most efficient form of energy production is the utilization of fat, which leads to the greatest increase in endurance. Any time you have to breathe through your mouth, or cannot carry on a conversation while exercising, you are burning sugar, not fat. You should never feel "wiped out" after exercising. Remember, the goal is to increase brain functioning and, consequently, productivity and vitality, not to beat yourself up physically.

Sometimes people have limitations that prevent them from doing certain types of exercise. I can relate to this. For example, I can't run. However, there is always some way you can move your body. How about a stationary bike, stepper, or treadmill? If this is not possible, yoga, tai chi, and chi gong are excellent forms of slow movement exercises. If you can't use your legs, use your arms. Take what the body gives you and work with it. I recently saw a senior citizen doing laps around a high school track using his walker. Now, that's determination!

Strive for an exercise routine of three to four days a week. Include strength training, and exercise each muscle group twice a week. Lean muscle mass is a primary indicator of good health. Muscles are also a storehouse of certain important nutrients, and muscle exercises help promote healthy hormone levels and stabilize blood sugar.

An exercise program can add as much as two hours of additional productive time to each day. The challenge is to start. If you are not exercising now, start with five minutes per day. If you are exercising, add five minutes to your routine. If your exercise routine is already long enough, look at how you can improve it. Less rest time between exercises might be an option.

I remember working out at a local YMCA when I was in my youth. I used to watch a particular group of guys sit and read the *Wall Street Journal* in the gym. Every once in a while one would get up and do something. At the other end of the spectrum was fitness expert Jack LaLanne. He not only did not rest at all between exercises, he would literally run through his whole routine, which was commonly over two hours.

The holistic model of health and disease is that you do not go from one side to the other overnight. It is a gradual process. In that broad middle ground, there are most often signs and symptoms, but not a clear-cut diagnosis. When there is a clear-cut diagnosis, it can be called a *disease*. If there is an imbalance in the body, with signs and symptoms, but no diagnosis or labels, it is a *dis-ease*.

Unfortunately, these signs and symptoms are ignored, or efforts are introduced to suppress symptoms as if they were the problem. This approach does not work to stop the progression toward a more serious dis-ease, and, many times, leads to more serious problems than the original complaints.

Most of what is done in health care is directed toward suppressing symptoms that are begging us to investigate what the manifestation of these alarms is really telling us.

In the case of the brain, there is a gradual decrease in mental performance. Problems usually start with memory loss and the inability to retrieve information. Difficulty focusing is also part of the process of decline. Multi-tasking becomes very difficult. Brain fatigue follows and reaction time drops.

What is behind this epidemic of lagging brain function? It appears to be multi-factorial, but the underlying cause of much brain distress is often known to be inflammation.

Inflammation in the brain is caused by free radical production. Free radicals are unstable molecules that create heat, which damages surrounding tissue. In the brain, the fat cells become affected. Since the brain is 60% fat, there is a lot of potential for inflammation. Free radicals can be triggered by the intake of rancid overheated oils and hydrogenated fats. These artificial fats will displace the natural fats, which is one of the reasons they're so harmful, and it is difficult to remove them from the body.

Using unhealthy fats and oils, as well as microwave cooking, can create what is called lipid peroxidation. The negative effects can destroy brain and nerve tissue and damage the part of the cell that makes energy, the mitochondria. These effects can last for quite some time and result in fatigue and decreased concentration. Fatigue is the main complaint today. There is good evidence that most of the time it starts in the brain, not the body. We will discuss unhealthy fats in more detail later in this chapter and throughout the book. Fatigue will be addressed in Chapter 2.

It is known that some chemicals are the most potent causes of free radical activity in the brain. Many of these chemicals are neurological toxins. These could include such things as pesticides, insecticides, cleaning agents, and food additives. Many chemicals affect neurotransmitters which are needed for cellular communication. These neurotransmitters include acetylcholine, which affects memory and learning, dopamine, which affects balance and fine motor movement, and serotonin, which affects moods and appetite control. Function can't take place without cellular communication. When cellular communication suffers, function immediately starts to decline.

Combining a toxic exposure to chemicals, with a body that lacks antioxidants, can have dire consequences. Antioxidants are needed to neutralize free radicals. One common reason for people's lack of antioxidants is the medications they are taking. Many common over-the-counter medications, as well as prescriptions drugs, can destroy needed antioxidants.

Brain problems and diseases are on the rise, and much of this dysfunction has inflammation as a root cause. Serious diseases, like Alzheimer's and Parkinson's, are on the rise at alarming rates. Alzheimer's is being called the autism of adults. 10% of the American population at the age of 65 already has Alzheimer's. At the current rate of incidence, by 2030, eight million Americans will have this debilitating disease. It alone is enough to devastate our health care system. The picture with Parkinson's disease is equally bleak.

There are also less serious brain problems that still affect lives, our economy, and put the future of our country in question. 14% of school age children are diagnosed with Attention Deficit Disorder. Depression, anxiety, and obsessive compulsive disorders count for some of the top selling prescription drugs today. Psychotropic drugs are the biggest growth market for the pharmaceutical industry, and some of the most expensive medicines.

Lab tests can be helpful to determine the inflammatory load an individual has. Particularly if you are forgetting things, stumbling over your words, or have difficulty in retrieving something from memory, it is recommended that further investigation be done.

Here are some good tests to screen for possible inflammation problems within the body and brain:

Oxidative Stress Test
Lipid peroxidation is an accurate marker for free radical activity in fatty tissue. Remember, the brain is mostly fat. This test measures the degree of free radical assault that is taking place and also the antioxidant defense status of the individual.

Homocysteine
Homocysteine is a normal by-product of the methylation cycle. This is the breakdown of the amino acid methionine in the body, which normally produces homocysteine, but the body should neutralize it very quickly. If it does not, homocysteine, as it builds up, is inflammatory and can damage arteries. High levels are one of the risk factors for developing Alzheimer's.

Good nutrition can neutralize the presence of homocysteine. It is not supposed to stick around long. Once it is produced, the body should neutralize it very quickly.

Elevated levels of homocysteine are known to cause cardiovascular disease by damaging arteries. The brain can be a target, with actual shrinkage a result, along with decreased hand-eye coordination. It can contribute to an increased risk of depression, Alzheimer's disease, Parkinson's disease, stroke, and cancer. When homocysteine is produced, certain nutrients are required to neutralize it. Vitamin B6 and B12, folic acid and magnesium are a few. Drugs are not the solution here.

C-Reactive Protein

C-Reactive Protein (CRP) is another inflammatory marker. It has long been known to increase the risk of cardiovascular disease, but can also mean there is inflammation in the brain. Recent research has shown that turmeric can be an effective remedy at lowering CRP.

Glutathione

Glutathione is one of the best markers for health there is. The higher the levels, generally the better level of wellness one has. It is a potent cellular antioxidant and one of the most powerful antioxidants there is. Glutathione can be taken orally or administered intravenously. Precursors to glutathione can be taken to help boost levels in the body. N-acetyl cysteine is one. Lipoic acid is another. There are two enzymatic processes necessary to synthesize glutathione. One is selenium dependent, and the other is riboflavin dependent. These are important nutrients if you want to increase glutathione in the body. Whey protein has also been shown to help increase glutathione levels.

Antigliadin Antibody Test

This test measures for gluten intolerance. It can be important, because effects of gluten intolerance can manifest globally, including in the brain. Imaging can display white spots on the brain, similar to multiple sclerosis. It is worth ruling out. This problem is so common that any sign of increased brain inflammation is enough reason to suggest a no-gluten diet and protocols to eliminate any residual peptide fragments that may still reside in the body from past ingestion.

The body stores what it can't eliminate, so it is also important to minimize our exposure to other harmful substances that can be brain blasters. Not exposing ourselves to mercury is essential. Get old silver fillings replaced by a dentist trained in proper removal techniques. Do not use aluminum cookware or deodorants that contain it. There are also cake mixes and non-dairy creamers that contain it. Avoid unnecessary vaccines. Flu shots are high in mercury, contain aluminum, and are known to increase one's risk of Alzheimer's disease.

Do not use toxic insecticides and chemicals inside your home. Even use outside the home has been shown to greatly increase the risk of Parkinson's disease. There are natural alternatives, but even if there weren't, is it worth the risk? Fluoride that is added to our water supplies is a known toxin. No, this chemical is not naturally found in the human body. It is known to have a negative effect on the brain and many other systems of the body, and is highly recommended you avoid it entirely.

If there is inflammation in the brain due to toxicity of chemicals, pesticides, or heavy metals, they will need to be eliminated to reverse this process. Detoxification of the brain also depends on the body's ability to handle and eliminate the offending substances.

When toxins are liberated from the tissues, they wind up at the liver, to go through its amazing detox system. Toxins can then be excreted either in the feces or urine. Lipoic acid, with its ability to cross the blood-brain barrier, is a great cellular and liver antioxidant and helps detoxify heavy metals, especially mercury. Lipoic acid is also a constituent of the citric acid cycle which produces ATP (energy), so a positive effect on one's energy levels is a common response. N-acetyl cysteine is another great de-toxifier, particularly aiding the liver. Cilantro and chlorella promote the excretion of mercury. Magnesium and selenium are two main minerals that help detoxify several chemicals as well as mercury. Calcium d-glucarate helps the glucuronidation detox pathway in the liver. This is the route that excess hormone and hormone mimickers, like certain pesticides and plastics, must go through in the liver to be eliminated from the body. If liver functioning is not adequate, the toxins will stay in the tissues. As you see, a healthy brain and body are very dependent on a healthy liver.

There are many nutritional foods that promote a healthy brain.

Berries, particularly blueberries, are at the top of the list. They are loaded with healthy substances like anthocyanins, which are beneficial to the cells and the nervous system. Blueberries have actually been shown to reverse signs of a declining brain.

Wild Alaskan salmon is another great food. It is loaded with healthy omega-3 fatty acids. No, farmed salmon does not count. It is not even close to being the same as the wild, natural fish. The Alaskan salmon have been shown to be very low in mercury contamination as well. It seems the closer to the main body of the United States the fish are harvested, the higher the levels of contamination.

Walnuts are good brain food and a great source of omega-3 fatty acids. Here is a clue. Break open a walnut. Ever see a picture of a brain? Doesn't it look similar? By the way, it is best to get whole walnuts, if you can, and crack them open just before you eat them. The nutrient and enzyme levels are higher that way.

Spinach is good brain food. It has also shown to reverse signs of brain aging. It is also a tonic to the kidneys, which is another big part of our detoxification system. Organic eggs are loaded with good fat and lecithin, a natural cholesterol mobilizer. Eggs are a rich source of choline, which the body uses to make the important neurotransmitter, acetylcholine, used for learning and memory.

Water is essential. The brain is adversely affected by as little as 10% dehydration. The body and brain need adequate water to function and detoxify.

To maintain a healthy brain, the following are some nutritional "don'ts", which should never be consumed in this lifetime. How some of these things were allowed into our food supply is a sad indictment of how politics and profits have taken precedence over the health of our people.

Here are items to avoid totally:

- Hydrogenated fats and oils
- Deli meats
- Fried foods
- Corn and soy oil
- Artificial sweeteners
- MSG
- Fluoride
- Artificial flavors and colors

Some of these may be regular staples in your diet, or perhaps they are hidden within ingredient labels you've never noticed. In either case, let's explore reasons why it is important to replace them with healthier choices.

Hydrogenated fats are fake fats. The hydrogenation process solidifies the natural fats and oils in foods to prevent separation. For example, open a jar of natural peanut butter and you will see the oil sitting on top that you stir in before eating. Open a jar of processed peanut butter and you will notice there is no visible oil on top. It is solid and "harder," closer to plastic than food. Eating this non-food does a number on your cell membranes. Cell membranes are made of lipids, and their quality is directly related to the fats in the diet. As the cell membranes become harder from the hydrogenated fats, they become less functional. A fluid membrane allows nutrients to get inside the cell and toxins to exit the cell. When that can't happen, the cell is in trouble.

Hydrogenation is done because it is cheap and prolongs shelf life, but do not count on it prolonging your life. Remember, the brain is loaded with healthy fat. Imagine if that fat was predominately hard, fake fat. Do you think that might have an effect on the brain? This stuff should not be in the food supply and in much of the world, outside the United States, it is not.

Deli meats are very hard to digest and have little nutritional benefit. They actually require the immune system to be activated to neutralize what the digestive system can't break down. White blood cells are dramatically and measurably increased after eating a hot dog, for example. That is an indication of poisoning, rather than nourishing, the body. It is also known that diabetes and colon cancer rates increase considerably in people who eat a lot of processed meats.

Rancid oils increase the amount of inflammation from lipid peroxidation. It is best not to fry foods, but when you must, use only good, natural oils (like extra-virgin olive or coconut oil) and do not use high heat.

Exitotoxins are called such because these chemicals can excite brain neurons to death. MSG, also known as monosodium glutamate, and NutraSweet ™ are two of the more popular ones. They are poisons to the brain and liver. Over 100 million pounds of MSG are used in fast food restaurants every year. NutraSweet ™ is found in over 6,000 products. Avoid these totally. There is no positive side to consuming these items.

Fluoride is a toxic waste that is added to much of the country's water supplies. The health-damaging effects of fluoride are enough to fill a book, but one such effect is its ability to lower one's IQ. As a side note, it was recently reported that much of the fluoride used in the U.S. is imported from China and is high in heavy metal contamination, which can also affect the brain negatively.

Nutritional supplements can be of great benefit to the brain. Here are several that can help make major improvements:

Coenzyme Q10
A necessary nutrient for energy production, with antioxidant and immune boosting capabilities.

Acetyl L-Carnitine

Helps with cellular detoxification, maintains nerve cell production, and has been shown to decrease Parkinson's risk (along with lipoic acid).

Phosphatidylserine

Promotes healthy cellular membranes, improves memory and increases the neurotransmitter acetylcholine.

Resveratrol

A potent antioxidant and helps oxygenate the brain. It also increases the anti-aging gene SIRT1, which decreases neurodegeneration and increases plasticity, which is the actual building of new nerve pathways, something science previously assumed wasn't possible.

Grape Seed Extract

Increases brain glutathione, the most potent antioxidant.

B Vitamins

Particularly B6, B12, and B3 are good for the nerves. B3 has been shown to be helpful in treating Alzheimer's disease.

DHA

An important fatty acid that is concentrated in the brain.

Lipoic Acid

Helps detoxify heavy metals and maintains nerve cell energy production. It is part of the citric acid cycle which makes ATP (energy) in the body.

L-Carnosine

A great anti-aging nutrient. Helps with nerve repair, increases synaptic activity in the brain's frontal cortex, and lessens stress-induced damage to the brain and kidneys from too much cortisol over a long period of time.

Beyond foods and nutrients, there are other components necessary for the brain to thrive. Here are some important ones:

- Movement with focus. Automatic movement without focus and attention do not provide the brain new information. Focus stimulates the growth of new nerve pathways. Doing movement slowly with focus is even more powerful.
- Learning new things is rocket fuel for the brain. The brain thrives on it. Taking classes, visiting new places, learning new recipes, and doing other exciting activities forms new brain patterns. New brain patterns equate to an increased sense of aliveness.
- Gentleness increases our vitality, awareness, and sensitivity.

- Excessive force does the opposite and leads to aches and pains.
- Diversity is needed to create new brain patterns. Doing things the same way all the time squeezes our vitality and restricts how we think and feel.

Our lifestyle habits affect our brain in a major way. Here are some tips that will create a vibrant brain:

- Exercise regularly. Exercise actually increases the number of mitochondria within our cells. This means our ability to make energy is enhanced. X-ray scans have proven that exercise increases circulation to the part of the brain that deals with learning and memory. Exercise can push back cognitive decline ten to fifteen years. It also promotes production of nerve pathway protection and improves neuron development and decreases cellular deterioration.
- Take drugs only when necessary for as short of a time as possible. Cognitive decline is the common denominator of all drugs, legal or illegal.
- Have fun. A childlike (not childish), playful attitude is good for our brains and immune systems.
- Get enough rest. Forty million Americans suffer from a sleep disorder. Americans also get 20% less sleep than people 100 years ago. Sleep deprivation decreases our cogni-

tive function and affects our nervous system similarly to alcohol. It can cause long-term damage to brain cells and does not allow repair to take place, since the body does most of its repair during sleep.

- Control your stress. This is a must. Whole books are written about the harmful effects of stress. It increases free radical production which causes inflammation and interferes with our body's efforts to make energy. Stress is toxic to our memory center of the brain and decreases the production of neurotransmitters, which are necessary for cellular communication.

Do something you love for your work. This is important. If that is not possible, do something you love while you do your work.

Surround yourself with beautiful music, colors, smells, and things that delight you. They will make you feel good and the brain loves it. Where you spend most of your time should be heaven to your senses.

chapter TWO

ENERGY IS EVERYTHING

Fatigue is epidemic. Today, it is the number one complaint that brings people to the doctor's office. Without energy, people spend most of their efforts just trying to get through the day. To truly have a vibrant, youthful life, abundant energy is a must. Why is having enough energy so rare?

There are physical and non-physical reasons for fatigue. It is important to note that everything counts. If fatigue is a major issue for you, as it is for the vast majority of people, then you are overdrawn on your energy bank account. There may be too many energy draining factors in your life and not enough energy enhancers. The "drainers" need to be identified and eliminated or changed.

The first step is awareness. The second step is taking action. Begin by asking yourself this question about what you eat and do, *"Does this _____ (fill in the blank) increase or decrease my energy?"*

Based on my years of clinical experience, there are nine main factors that will drain your energy:

Undiagnosed infections.

Many people have chronic infections they are not aware of that are dragging them down. The infection can be viral, bacterial, parasitic, yeast or fungal, to name a few. It takes a lot of energy for the body to function and cope with this stress at the same time. The body gets depleted of its vitality, as the immune system is under constant pressure. Many times there are indications of low level infection that show on routine blood tests but go ignored. Doctors usually focus on acute, severe infection indicators because they are trained to focus on disease diagnosis. That is the nature of their education. This problem of missed infections is more common than most realize.

Immune system depletion

When the immune system is exhausted, you are exhausted. There are multiple components to the immune system. With over 70% of it actually in the vicinity of the intestines, digestive problems can stimulate our immunity. For example, when the small intestine becomes irritated, it can actually leak food into circulation, causing a common problem called *leaky gut syndrome*. To deal with this leakage, the immune system produces an antibody that attaches to the food, which is now a foreign invader to the body, much like a virus or bacteria. This suppresses the immune system by wearing it down. If it happens after every meal, people will remark how fatigued they feel.

Some reach the point where they dread having to eat because they are well aware of the consequences. When an antibody attaches to an antigen, this is referred to as a circulating immune complex. It will eventually become lodged in the joints or tissues if the body can't eliminate it. This is a major cause of inflammation, whether it is called arthritis, fibromyalgia or something else.

Other major players in the immune system are the spleen and thymus. The spleen is primarily concerned with general immunity. It also has other functions, like aiding digestion, controlling mucous production, and dealing with blood quality. According to Chinese medicine, the spleen is where energy is produced. It is only logical then that, if the spleen is exhausted, energy levels will suffer.

The thymus gland deals with specific immunity. The thymus is the "university" of the immune system, making specific antibodies for the particular antigens that the body is fighting off. It also makes natural killer cells, which are vitally important for keeping us healthy. Thymus stress also affects energy levels greatly. Mushrooms can have a potent tonic effect on the thymus gland. Shiitake, reishi, and maitake varieties are excellent boosters to the immune system.

Sluggish thyroid

The thyroid controls our basal metabolic rate. It also affects our moods and motivation levels, as well as our energy. I mention the thyroid because it is commonly found to need help. Blood test results may or may not indicate an imbalance. Thyroid blood tests are not the most sensitive of blood tests and they miss a lot of thyroid issues that need treating. If the blood test is abnormal, then the imbalance is usually severe. Many times, I will see test results at the end of normal ranges. This normal reading, probably set by an insurance company, does not necessarily coincide with the actual state of one's thyroid. The physical exam I provide for my patients incorporates analyzing reflex responses in the nervous system and displays if the gland is under stress, regardless of the lab numbers.

Even if the patient is taking a thyroid hormone, the gland can still be, and usually is, out of balance. Supplementing with the hormone can change the numbers, but does not resolve why the thyroid is not making enough hormone on its own. *"Why is the thyroid not making thyroid hormone?"* is the question that should be asked.

There are certain ingredients required for the thyroid to function optimally, including minerals like iodine, zinc, manganese, and selenium. The amino acid L-tyrosine and essential fatty acids are also needed.

Inflammation

Inflammatory conditions are at the root of all disease processes. Before the dis-ease was diagnosed, there most likely was inflammation running rampant for a long time. Inflammation causes fatigue as well as pain. The lab tests for discerning inflammation mentioned in Chapter 1 also apply here.

Toxicity

In my experience, toxicity is one of the top causes of fatigue. It can come from internal sources, like undigested food, or external sources, like drugs and other foreign toxins. Too much undigested food within the body does the same thing in the intestines it would do in a garbage can. This becomes a prime environment for "garbage eaters," like bacteria and parasites. In my opinion, every adult needs digestive help. Using the appropriate digestive enzymes will help deliver more nutrition from food and decrease the amount of waste buildup that has not been adequately broken down. A certified Enzyme Therapist can be of great assistance here, of which I am one. A small number of professionals are trained in this area. The Loomis Institute in Madison, Wisconsin has a comprehensive list of therapists on their website http://www.loomisinstitute.com/.

There are many external sources of toxins, but the biggest threats come from pesticides, chemicals, and heavy metals. There are literally thousands of chemicals in our food supply and drinking water. It is impossible to totally avoid pesticides, with over a billion pounds being used in the U.S. annually. Even if we are not eating them in food, we are breathing them. A number of years ago, breast milk samples tested in natives in a remote area of New Guinea all had pesticide residues in them. It took two days for researchers to hike through New Guinea to reach these people, who did not even know what pesticides were, so they certainly weren't using them. What do you think our chance is to be free of these toxins? Right. We have zero chance of being unscathed by this assault on humanity.

Remember, as we discussed in Chapter 1, what the body can't eliminate, it stores. One of the favorite places for the storage of hormones and pesticides is in the breast tissue. Hormones and hormone mimickers will go to the nearest estrogen receptor sites if they are not eliminated by the liver. Those sites are located in the breast tissue. Over time, lumps can form and cancer risk increases.

Drugs are also a major source of toxicity today. With over 50% of the population regularly taking prescription drugs, this is noteworthy. The average adult takes six drugs per year. At age 65, the average American is on 13 drugs. All drugs, both legal and illegal, have toxic side effects.

One of those effects is fatigue. In fact, the majority of the top selling prescription medicines list fatigue as a possible consequence of their use.

The programming today is to view drugs as the way to health. While there is a time and place for drugs, it is illogical to look at these synthetic compounds as the way to get healthier. The body does not thrive on drugs, which work by blocking metabolic processes, instead of supporting them. For people whose mindset is that drugs equal health, they generally notice their daily list of pills to take gets longer over time, and their quality of life gets worse. Cognitive decline takes place as the toxicity from the drugs builds up. It is not unusual to notice the slowing down of mental ability and even personality changes. A classic example was Elvis Presley. As he used more and more drugs (all legal), the people around him remarked how bizarre his behavior became.

A widespread example is the annual flu vaccine. People ask me all the time, *"Do you think I should get a flu shot?"* My answer is always no, mainly because of the toxicity of the shot. While the efficacy of the shot can be debated, the toxic levels of mercury and other chemical additives override any possible benefit of the vaccine. There is nothing good about mercury or aluminum being injected into the human body. The potential risk for diseases like Alzheimer's goes way up with these poisons being put into the body. Vaccinations are not the only source of these toxins, but the sheer numbers being given today make them a major source.

So, what can we do? First, we can aid the body's efforts to detoxify these poisons. Most of that effort should be directed toward supporting the liver. Supplements, like calcium d-glucarate, can be helpful. The detox pathway in the liver that breaks down hormones and hormone mimickers, like pesticides, is the glucuronidation pathway. Calcium d-glucarate supports the liver's efforts here and is probably one of the best breast cancer preventions there is. There are other nutrients that support liver detoxification. Selenium, N-acetyl cysteine, safflower and milk thistle are a few. We can also make more of an effort to eat organically grown foods. One of the biggest reasons that natural, organic foods are recommended is the absence of chemicals.

Another type of toxicity that can be just as damaging to our health and energy are toxic emotions. Emotions, like hate, resentment, hostility, jealousy, and pessimism are toxic, draining and release chemicals within the body that cause dis-ease. These emotions do nothing to harm anybody but you. They need to be released and replaced with positive emotions.

For any perceived negative event in your past, it is important to reframe it, look for the lesson, and have a sense of gratitude for it. There is always a lesson to learn. Focusing on the lesson and moving forward is more constructive than staying stuck in emotions that run your life and hold you back. Releasing these toxic emotions will create a lightness and increased vitality beyond what you can imagine at this point.

Toxic relationships are also draining. They need to be changed or eliminated. List the people in your life and rate them with a plus if they energize you and a minus if they drain you. Then make a second list of the names with minuses, and leave space between each name. Next to each person, list what you do not like about the relationship. What characteristics of each person bother you? Is it possible you might share these same qualities? Maybe these people are mirrors of things you need to work on. Perhaps you are tolerating things that are unacceptable to you, yet, rather than taking action, you berate yourself for not confronting the situation.

I do believe that sometimes the best course of action is to eliminate some people from our lives. They might even be family members in some cases. It can be difficult, but limiting your exposure to the negativity of others can be liberating and energy enhancing.

The key point here is to surround yourself with people who are uplifting. You can't help but be influenced by the people around you. Your reference group is one of the biggest determining factors in how successful your life will be. Those who choose to always rain on your parade can do so somewhere else. Wayne Dyer used to say, *"Nobody has the right to ruin my day,"* and he made sure nobody did. He did not give them that power. Good advice, in my opinion.

Nutrient depletion

The body needs certain raw materials in order to make energy. Some important nutrients are magnesium, B vitamins, with a particular emphasis on folic acid, lipoic acid, essential fatty acids, L-carnitine, and coenzyme Q10. A shortage of any of these nutrients can have negative consequences in the energy department.

Here are some of the reasons these nutrients are so important and a few ways the body can become depleted.

These days, many people seem to need magnesium, a mineral used in about three hundred and fifty metabolic pathways. It is a major factor for energy, as shown in these two key processes. First, the beginning step in sugar metabolism is magnesium dependent. A diet high in sugar and refined carbohydrates causes depletion of nutrients and minerals, particularly magnesium.

Second, magnesium helps rid the body of acidity from exercise exertion, thus aiding recovery time. Magnesium also helps muscles relax, another reason it aids recovery time. Endurance athletes are shown to have increased their performances by up to 30% by adding magnesium, along with potassium.

A magnesium deficiency can have severe consequences. Since cancer cells are acidic, and magnesium alkalizes cells, it only stands to reason cancer cells are deficient in magnesium. Magnesium can also become depleted with dysbiosis, which is an imbalance in the ecological terrain of the intestines, where there are not enough friendly bacteria in the intestinal flora. An overgrowth of too much bad bacteria, yeast, or fungus is common in the intestines. Too many refined foods in the diet, too much caffeine, and excessive alcohol use can contribute to both problems.

B vitamin depletion can cause fatigue in the following ways:

- Vitamin B1, or thiamin, is extremely important for energy production. The first step in converting glucose to energy inside the cell is B1 dependent. It also has a stimulating effect on the nervous system and can help strengthen the heart as well as the bladder and kidneys. A high sugar diet and many diuretics deplete B1 levels.

- Vitamin B6 is necessary for nerve health and protein metabolism. Neurological problems, cold hands and feet, stiffness in the fingers, and hormonal problems could manifest with this deficiency. B6 is depleted with a diet high in processed foods and certain prescription drugs, with birth control pills being among the worst offenders. For B6 to be used by the body, it must be converted in the liver to pyridoxal-5'–phosphate (P5P). If there are glitches in the liver preventing that process, results won't happen. The active form is available from a few companies to bypass reliance on the liver.

- Several years ago, Harper's Biochemistry Review called folic acid (B9) the number one nutritional deficiency in the United States. The nervous system requires folic acid. Shortage during pregnancy can lead to neural tube defects or cleft palates. It also helps with protein metabolism and is a gene protectant, making it a cancer preventative. A lack of folic acid can cause anemia, depression, and fatigue.

- Vitamin B12 depletion can lead to B12 anemia, which causes fatigue. B12 is necessary for nerve health and low levels can contribute to dementia. An orthopedic test called the Shillings Test, has long been used as a diagnostic indicator of muscular sclerosis (MS) and has also been found to be indicative of a B12 deficiency. It can mimic the neurological symptoms of MS. Again, a refined diet can cause a deficiency, but so can digestive problems in the stomach. Stomach medications and antacids can also be a factor in depleting the body's stores of vitamin B12.

- Lipoic acid is a constituent of the citric acid cycle, which makes adenosine triphosphate (ATP) for energy in the body. Lipoic acid is a precursor to glutathione synthesis, which is the most potent antioxidant in the body. It is a heavy metal chelator and has the ability to cross the blood-brain barrier, making it a great brain detoxifier. It is a potent liver support and rejuvenator.

- Essential fatty acids, or EFAs, are called such because they are essential to make energy, particularly for endurance. The body is most efficient when it is burning fat most of the time for energy. The fat available in the body for this process is directly related to the quality of fat consumed in the diet. Natural fats are necessary and healthy. Besides being needed for energy, our brain, thyroid, and hormonal system require good fat sources for their functioning. These good fats are becoming increasingly difficult to get unless you make a conscious effort to consume them. Natural fats are found in unaltered foods, like eggs, avocados, wild salmon, nuts, and seeds.

As I previously mentioned in Chapter 1, the unnatural or trans fats so often found in food products are not only unhealthy, they displace good fats and take a long time to get out of the body. Some unnatural fats and hydrogenated oils to watch out for are in margarine, processed peanut butter, mayonnaise, pastries, and some breads. A body loaded with trans fats in its cell membranes cannot possibly function optimally. Trans fats are hard, and that is exactly what they do to the cell walls, decreasing fluidity and, by doing so, hindering the cell's functioning. Getting nutrients inside the cell becomes as difficult as getting the toxins out. Remember, you are *never* better off with unnatural, fake foods.

L-carnitine carries the essential fatty acids inside the mitochondria of the cell where energy is made. It also helps transport toxins out of the cell. L-carnitine can be taken before a workout to enhance energy, or it can be taken ten minutes before meals to aid with the burning of fat.

Coenzyme Q10 is a powerful antioxidant and is important to all cellular function. The widespread use of pharmaceutical drugs is a primary reason for coenzyme Q10 depletion. It is normally manufactured in the liver, so liver issues can deplete it. Certain medications, particularly statin drugs to lower cholesterol, can deplete the body of this coenzyme, which can cause weakness in all muscles, including the heart. I will discuss more health repercussions in Chapter 4, in the first myth "The lower your cholesterol is, the better off you are" and in Chapter 5, in the "Cardiovascular Disease" section, under remedies for common ailments.

Tiredness

Tiredness is common. Many people simply do not get enough rest. Americans work more and take less time off than in any other industrialized country. They also get about 20% less sleep than 100 years ago. Try to get at least eight hours of sleep four days a week.

My advice is to take the time to recharge your batteries or eventually your body may force you to take the time off. It may come gradually or suddenly as low back pain, an illness or perhaps an injury. Take some time for yourself now to reinvigorate your vitality. What do you enjoy? Start there and do more of it. Take long weekends off. I recommend you start with at least one three-day weekend a month, and then go to one long weekend every second or third week. I can't emphasize this enough. It is an essential ingredient to good health and being a highly functioning human being.

Uncontrolled stress

To keep your energy up, you must learn how to control stress, or it will control you. Stress is draining. Often, it is caused by worry, which

I will cover in more detail in Chapter 3 and throughout the book. Stress usually becomes a degenerative, vicious cycle. When we are feeling stressed, we usually partake in habits that are stress-relieving in the short-term, but actually stimulate the stress response even more in the long-term. For example, it is common for people to eat more sugar when they are feeling stressed, drink more coffee or alcohol, skip exercise, or not get adequate rest. None of these things are solution oriented.

Most stress comes from feeling a lack of control. We get frustrated about things we feel we can't change. That is a total waste of energy. We need to get in touch with what is changeable and take action. Action is the antidote to stress. If you are not sure exactly what the best course of action is, take action of any kind for a short-term remedy. That could be something simple like starting an easy, regular exercise routine, cleaning out your closets, or fixing things that have been broken for some time. If we focus on the solutions, we will find them. Remember, if you feel you need support, it is always OK to ask for help.

If the stressor is not changeable, you need to change your perception of it. Reframe it and look for the positive in it. There is yin and yang in everything, even in a seemingly negative situation. Look for the good and open yourself up to what you can — and need to — learn from it. The situation is a teacher and it appeared for your benefit, just like the negative relationships with people in your life mentioned in the previous chapter. I know that is a tough concept, but many times, people will remark later that a particular stressful situation turned out to be the best thing that ever happened to them.

Physically, stress affects your adrenal glands. These glands pump out a stress hormone called cortisol. That is a very good thing if you are in a dangerous situation and need to act fast to save your life. However, cortisol being continually secreted is not a good thing. An ongoing fight or flight response is not healthy. It does a lot of damage to the body and brain. It suppresses the immune system, creates inflammation, causes pain, makes the body acidic, and can cause high blood pressure, hypoglycemia and even diabetes. Cortisol literally burns out the brain, causing continual excitation and inflammation that will hinder memory and learning.

Yes, stress can even make your mind less sharp. Eventually, the adrenal glands can become exhausted. When they wear down, low energy is definitely a side effect. Your efficiency goes further down as you have blood sugar swings, which can create dizziness and brain fog. Even exercising makes you feel worse when your adrenal glands are depleted.

The way out of this downward degenerative spiral is, of course, to deal with the stressful stimuli, and support the adrenals instead of continually whipping them. The best course of action is to see a practitioner of natural or functional medicine, skilled in assessing your specific needs. An easy way to begin at home is by getting off the stimulants and start eating whole, natural foods.

Adrenal exhaustion is one of the most common causes of unexplained fatigue in my opinion, and is rarely diagnosed correctly. There are a number of ways to tonify the adrenals, with the severity of the adrenal exhaustion being an important factor. Generally, supplementing with a B complex can be helpful and B5 (pantothenic acid) is especially beneficial to the brain. Siberian ginseng tonifies the adrenals, as does American ginseng. Licorice can be helpful. Ashwaganda can also be helpful, especially if a calming effect to the nervous system is needed. Rhodiola is also an excellent herbal tonic for the adrenals.

Living without a purpose

Another reason for a lack of energy is simply a lack of enthusiasm and living without a purpose. Most people are not excited about their lives or what they do for a living. They are occupied with just getting through the day. This uninspired existence is tiring. Since everything is made of energy, including us, it is obvious that there is not a lack of energy in the universe. However, just existing without a real purpose for our lives dis-connects us from the universal source of energy. Our plug is pulled, and then we have to rely on willpower to do our daily "work."

Many people are stressed because they are not doing what they love and feel trapped. It is esti-mated that 75% of Americans dislike their jobs immensely. It is no wonder we have such an ad-dicted society. People are trying to numb their feelings of unhappiness and the feeling of "Is this all there is?" There is no coincidence that most heart attacks happen on Monday mornings at work, particularly after a long weekend or vacation. People tell themselves things like, "*I don't want to be here,*" or "*Get me out of here.*" Your body believes every word you say, so these statements become self-fulfilling prophecies.

It is important to be on fire with your work. So, how do you improve the situation if you do not like your job? There are a couple of approaches to this. One is to find what you love to do, and figure out how to make a living doing it. The al-ternative is to do something you love while you do your work. This will help keep your energy up. As Dr. John DeMartini says,

"Link everything you do to your purpose and that will keep you constantly motivated and inspired."

This true story comes to mind. A gentleman was going to his room on an upper floor of a large hotel, and he realized he did not have his room key. Rather than go all the way down to the front desk, he went looking for the housekeeper on the floor. When he approached the room she was in, he heard the most beautiful singing. He apologized for interrupting her and asked for her assistance. He complimented her singing and stated she must really like her job, to be doing it in such a joyful manner. She replied she really did not like her job that much, but she loved to sing. That's a good example of doing what you love while you do your job.

Make the decision to change, and start taking steps to follow your passion. If you do not know what you love to do, find others who have found their passions, and work alongside them. Their enthusiasm will be contagious, and being around that energy will help you find what you love. Another option is to quit a job you are not happy with, and that will force you to make immediate changes. If you do not want to quit, then do what you love while at your current job, until you find the job you love.

We love to be around and watch people follow their passions. Many great athletes and entertainers fit into this category, and we will pay quite a bit of money for the opportunity to watch them do what they do. Why? Because they are passionate about what they do. We can feel it, and it makes us feel better. One of my favorite entertainers is singer and piano player Tom Bopp. If you have never heard of him, it is because he is not playing to sold-out auditoriums. He has been playing at the Wawona Hotel in Yosemite for 30 years. It is mesmerizing to watch him play one request after another (a lot of show tunes) and interact with the audience for hours at a time. He's truly following his passion and having a great time doing it.

Keep in mind that your purpose is not just an accomplishment. It is something you live for. Start setting goals that move you forward, so you can mark the passage of time with clarity. Both long-term and short-term goals are necessary to keep you inspired, and they can and should be linked to your purpose. Your purpose is what gives great significance to your achievements. Goals are necessary ingredients, but without a greater purpose, goals are harder to achieve and have less charge attached to them. Keith Leon, best-selling author of, *Who Do You Think You Are? Discover the Purpose of Your Life* says,

> *"Everything you need to know is already within you.
> You are the answer you have been looking for."*

Go within, and ask yourself these three important questions:

- Who am I?
- What is my purpose?
- Why am I here?

As these answers are eventually revealed to you, you will truly be reborn to a life that is intrinsically inspiring and energizing.

chapter THREE

STOP WORRYING,
START LIVING

Worry is one of the biggest roadblocks to maintaining, or regaining, a youthful life. It is not possible to have a well-balanced mental attitude and think with absolute clarity, when we are absorbed in worry. Worry is a destructive state of mind that causes mental distress.

If you are worried about something you can immediately resolve, then take action and remedy the situation. If, for example, you thought you left the stove on at home, go back and check it, or call someone else to do it. In either case, this is a legitimate concern and should be dealt with as soon as possible.

However, that is not the type of worry that runs most people's lives. What happens with most are ongoing emotional charges of apprehension, fear, anxiety or regret. There is nothing positive about having your life ruled by negativity. There is an old African proverb that says, *"If there is no enemy within, the enemy outside can do you no harm."* Worry is an enemy that prevents us from living vibrantly.

Most people are worried about what might happen in the future or happened in the past. Either way, it prevents you from living in the present. What gets missed is *today,* and today is all you have. To worry about the past or something you fear will happen in the future is a total waste of time and energy. Studies have shown that 30% of the time people are worried about things that have already happened. That is called sawing sawdust. Learn from it and move on. It is impossible to go back and change it. It is possible to change our perception of the situation, however, which is necessary sometimes to help us move on.

In other situations, 40% of the time people are worried about things that most likely will never happen in the future. Again, worrying keeps people from living today, and will not do anything to secure an ideal future outcome. People mistake worry for action. It is not. Quite the opposite is true. Worry has a paralyzing affect that prevents constructive action.

In 4% of situations, people worry over things about which nothing can be done. All the worry in the world won't change it. Can you think of a bigger waste of energy? 10% of worries are about petty matters that do not make any difference one way or another. This is called looking hard for something to worry about. And finally, 4% of worries are actually about situations that can be changed. So work on the solution, rather than just worrying about the problem.

Here is what most people's worries look like:

- 40% of people's worries are about things that will never happen.

- 30% are about things that happened in the past.
- 12% are useless worries about health.
- 10% are about petty things that do not matter.
- 4% are about things that can't be changed.
- 4% are about things that can actually be changed.

Is it any wonder why worry is called "the foolish American pastime"?

The effects of worry are many, but the main effects keep us from being in the present, so we are literally missing out on life, living like robots, under constant physical stress. Stress is a slow degenerative process, like dying from a thousand paper cuts. The continual buildup of many, small stressors that we habitually worry about, creeps up on us. Most are not even aware that it has taken over our lives. As Churchill put it, *"It's the broken shoelaces that destroy men's lives."*

After the worrying begins, and takes hold, the physical complaints will eventually manifest. Even the Mayo Clinic has stated that out of 15,000 patients with stomach disorders, four out of five had no physical basis. Nobel Prize winner Dr. Alexis Carel put it this way, *"Businessmen who do not know how to fight worry, die young."* This effect is not just limited to businessmen. Worry is water torture. It is the constant drip, drip, drip that drives people insane.

"The greatest mistake physicians make is to attempt to cure the body without curing the mind." — Plato

It has been said that worry and stress are responsible for more disease than all the germs on Earth. Worry disorganizes the whole body and disturbs the mind to the point it cannot effectively run the body. Eventually, the will becomes paralyzed. Stress comes from the belief you have no control over a particular situation. As long as you hold this perception, the stress response continues.

Worry causes stress and can create the following responses in the body:

- Decreased nutrient absorption
- Decreased oxygen to the gut
- Four times less blood flow to the gut
- Decreased enzymatic output in the gut
- Loss of vitamins, minerals, calcium and sodium
- Agitation of the brain region that controls short-term memory
- Liver and kidney stress as cortisol builds up

The physical effects of worry cause:

- High blood pressure
- Heart failure
- Insomnia
- Hormone imbalances
- Immune suppression
- Intestinal disorders (irritable bowel syndrome)

- Weight problems
- Hypoglycemia and diabetes

Dr. Solposki wrote a book called *Why Zebras Don't Get Ulcers*. Zebras are not under chronic stress. They mobilize their fight or flight response when running away from a lion. That is what the stress hormone cortisol is supposed to do, help the zebra save its life. This same hormone helps human beings when they're stressed. If the zebra survives and escapes from the lion, it will then dissipate the built up energy from its life-saving attempt. It will go through various gyrations with its body that help eliminate this pent up energy from the built up trauma.

People do not dissipate this energy. Instead, they generally suppress it. Carrying around a stressful memory, a trauma that is being relived every day, literally destroys people from the inside out. These locked-in negative emotions must be dealt with. It is important to look for the opportunity that is presented in every perceived negative situation, and look for the lesson that is always there.

Once, I observed a man totally lose control in a video store because the movie he wanted, which the store guaranteed to be in stock or they would provide a free rental, was not available. The man's temper exploded because he wanted only what he came in for. This could have become a very dangerous situation — over a movie. When stress gets to that point of overwhelm, it really makes people stupid. All of the blood and energy goes to the reptilian part of the brain for "fight or flight." He was so overwhelmingly out of control that the stress changes in his body were visible.

He lashed out as if he were facing a life-threatening situation (again, over a movie). This is not an exaggeration.

Think of instances in your own life when you have observed similar situations. When people react from the survival part of the brain all the time, toxic chemicals are released into their blood, which raises their blood pressure, suppresses their immune system, and creates severe acidity in their bodies that can cause pain and dis-ease. The blood can become so toxic just one drop injected into a rabbit can kill it. Stress hormones fry the short-term memory center of the brain, create intestinal inflammation, which can cause ulcers, Crohn's disease or ulcerative colitis, put a toxic load on the liver and also negatively affect the kidneys.

Ever watch people at an airport when their planes are delayed? Some will go bonkers. They will scream and shout at the gate attendants. What effect do you think that behavior has on the schedule of the airplane? Absolutely none. The plane will get there when it gets there. What a waste of time and energy to react so negatively to something totally out of your control. Again, the feeling of not having any control is what causes most of people's stress. It has been my observation that those who always try to control other people and events have the least amount of self-control.

Here are some positive ways to deal with the stress response.

Exercise regularly

Not excessive, but regular, moderate exercise is a great way to let go of worry and stress.

Get enough rest

Worry is depleting. Take time to recharge your batteries, and focus on something inspiring and motivating, which has you in a state of gratitude and appreciation.

Eat to nourish your body

Do not eat for stress relief or just for pleasure. Eat with the awareness of how to serve your body temple with the proper eating habits. By the way, nourishing food usually tastes better and is more pleasurable than the junk you used to eat.

Meditate

Meditation is an excellent way to deal with the stress caused by worry. Sit in silence. If this is new to you, it is usually difficult to quiet the mind in the beginning. A simple way to begin is to focus on your breathing. Focus on the breath in and the breath out. That will keep your mind from wandering and is a great starting point.

Conquer your stress

There are many resources to help with conquering worry and stress. You might want to check out the Heart Math Institute and the Sedona Method. Many other resources are available, but these are two good ones. Meditation, counseling and various types of body work can also be helpful, such as the **Feldenkrais Method**® and Neuro Emotional Technique (NET), founded by Dr. Scott Walker in the San Diego area.

Why are some people so intent on constantly worrying? One possible explanation is that it is learned behavior. If you were raised in a home where one or both parents were worriers, you could be emulating that behavior without realizing it. You became "wired" to worry due to this childhood programming. You are just copying what is familiar, and, unless you make a conscious effort to undo this programming, you will automatically revert back to it every time certain triggers are activated.

Worry can result because of a past trauma that had a profound negative effect. It is possible to frequently worry that it might happen again. There can also be things that stimulate our senses so memories are brought up that are the "on" switch for worry to begin. This trigger could be something that is said on the television news, lyrics to a song or a particular smell. Smells go directly to the part of the brain called the amygdala, which is also where memories are stored. Seeing a particular place where a traumatic event took place can trigger worry as well.

Just the sight of the location can cause worry about a repeat of what happened. That happened to me a couple of years ago. I had a flat tire on a particularly busy freeway with very little shoulder room. There I was, after dark, about two feet off the shoulder with heavy traffic zooming along at 70 plus miles per hour. Here cars would veer to the right to merge onto another freeway. It would have been easy for another driver to not realize my vehicle was on the shoulder, or not moving, and crash into me. There was no safe place to wait for the emergency vehicle to arrive. Everything worked out as I had the tire changed and got on my way, but the wait seemed like forever and I was very anxious about being in such a dangerous spot. I noticed afterwards that every time I drove by that same location, I felt fearful about getting a flat tire and very nervous. Even now, two years later, I do not drive by there without that memory coming up.

With some people, however, worry can be a habit and even an addiction. Because worry can cause a stress response which stimulates cortisol secretion by the adrenal glands, some get to where they thrive on the drug effect. In fact, some have a hard time functioning without it. Baby boomers are notorious for this pattern. Perhaps that's because during World War II many of their parents were born into scarcity and, consequently, this time of life was stressful for everyone. As I mentioned earlier, some people mistake worry for action. Somehow, they think they are doing some good by worrying, and it will really make a difference. It won't. The only difference will be to the health of the worrier's mind and body.

Another reason people worry engages what is called an *upper limit problem*. This is described by Brian Tracy in his excellent book, *Maximum Achievement*. The basic premise is that we have a thermostat setting for where we want to be in life. This is our comfort zone. Worry is a mechanism people use so they do not exceed the upper limit of their comfort zone. Most worry has nothing to do with what a person thinks it does. Instead, it functions to keep us miserable and unhappy. For example, most money problems in a marriage usually have very little to do with money. The amazing thing is that people do this to themselves. They have their own finger on their misery button, and they use it all the time without realizing they are doing so.

What is really behind an upper limit problem? According to Tracy, there are a couple of underlying basic beliefs that exist to prevent us from expanding into our greatness; they both utilize worry as a tool to prove ourselves right about our limitations. It is all about stopping the flow of good into our lives.

The first erroneous belief is the feeling of being fundamentally flawed. We feel there is something wrong with us. If we believe there is something wrong with us, we can't possibly believe we deserve great things. If we try to hold the thought that we do deserve to be massively successful, but at a deep level we really believe the opposite, the result is cognitive dissonance. When we try to hold two opposing thoughts at the same time, the battle in our minds must be resolved in one of two ways. Either we will return to our old pattern, or let go and release the old limiting belief. If we do not challenge the false belief, we will always go back to its hypnotic hold on us.

The fear of failure exists along with feeling flawed. The fear is that, even if you stretched yourself, it would never be good enough. It keeps us playing it safe, and that means playing small. It is a belief that failure goes along with being flawed. We believe it is who we are, failures, and flawed ones at that.

Of course, this is all in error. Failure has nothing to do with who we are, and we are not flawed. We need to embrace failure as a step to success. Successful people fail more than unsuccessful people because they try more things. Here is the difference, however. First, successful people do not look at the failure as permanent, and second, they learn from it. It is actually part of the path to success. It is a very different way to look at events and prevents the winners from quitting. They will not be convinced otherwise.

Another basic belief that holds us back and keeps us in our comfort zone is the fear of disloyalty and abandonment. The worry is that, if people expand and break new ground, they will end up alone, be disloyal to their roots and be forced to leave people they love behind. This creates feelings of guilt (as crazy as it sounds). This will show up in people's lives when they follow big breakthroughs with sabotaging behavior. This is also common for people who make a lot of money, then act in ways that cause them to lose it, or something similar. This is a very common scenario.

Many people believe increased success actually equals more of a burden. This can be taken to the extreme, that one's very existence is a burden to the world, his parents, siblings, and others. This is an effective technique to keep beating ourselves down. To worry more about doing well, than doing poorly, would seem illogical to anybody outside the situation. As the saying goes, you can't see the picture if you're in the frame.

Fear of outshining others is another common and illogical worry. If you shine too much, you might make others look bad or cause them to feel badly about themselves, which would result in making you feel bad about yourself, so you become hesitant to display your gifts to the world. This is very common with gifted children. They will hold their talents in check or downplay their successes, even to the point of being negative about them. They respond to compliments with negative comments about their performances. They would display suffering to elicit empathy and sympathy responses rather than jealousy. Jealousy can be a controlling, manipulative response that is quite powerful if allowed to be, and these children are aware of it from an early age.

All of these actions are particularly noticeable when things are going well. Our auto-regulatory thermostat will kick in to block the flow of positive in our life. Worry serves that purpose. Most worry has nothing to do with reality. Chronic worry is an addiction. Sometimes we hit the jackpot when our worry proves us right and justifies more worry. This is a most destructive, degenerative process that is not conducive to our being efficient, productive people.

Like all addictions, at some level we feel a need to worry because there is some payoff to the process. It makes us feel better at some level in the short-term. The problem is the payoff is not constructive. The best remedy is to eliminate the addiction. With awareness and helpful tools, this is definitely a doable objective.

The following are eight empowering action steps to eliminate worry:

1. Write down precisely what you are worrying about. You must become aware of the problem to do anything about it. This journaling exercise will help you to get in touch with it. Sometimes it is obvious, but not always. Spend some time doing this. Most worry is done automatically without thinking about the problem or analyzing it. What exactly do you feel is going to happen, and why are you worrying about it?

2. What can you do about it? Go back to your list of worries, and categorize each one. Determine where each one fits in. Is this a past or future kind of worry? Is it something you can actually do something about? If it is, then start an action plan to work on it. If it is not, then a different approach needs to be taken, like releasing, forgiving, or accepting. Begin by coming to terms with where each worry fits and considering what you can do about it, if anything.

3. Decide what to do. Get specific, and decide what your options are. This step will put you in control of the situation and decrease your stress levels immediately, since the stress response is directly correlated to the degree you feel a lack of control. I recommend writing down all that comes to mind regarding action steps you can take and then prioritizing the list. What actions give you the most return on your investment? Number your list with #1 being the highest priority, #2 being less than #1, etc. If you have more than one #1, is it reasonable that you can do all of them? If not, reprioritize all the #1s and start with the one that will make the biggest immediate difference.

4. Start immediately. Do it NOW. Nothing will change until you take action and start. If you do not start, then you simply are not serious and are actually content where you are. You know that is not true, so why not begin right away? You may think the payoff of waiting is worth it, but that is a lie you are telling yourself. When you quit lying to yourself, you will take a giant leap toward real authenticity, and your life will change.

5. Get completely occupied doing something constructive. Even if you do not have your action steps prioritized perfectly, by being busy you will not have time to worry. Remember, an idle mind will usually revert back to its previous programming. Do not trust your mind to itself.

6. Do not sweat the small stuff. Life is too short. Most differences between people, marriages that fall apart, even assaults and worse, have their roots in trivialities that became exaggerated. Do not let your mind take something small and run with it. Worrying is simply too expensive to your health, vitality, efficiency, and vibrancy.

On the slope of Long's Peak in Colorado, there was an ancient gigantic tree that had been struck by lightning fourteen times and survived some of the harshest winters. It was so old; it was a seedling when Columbus landed. What destroyed this tree was a tiny beetle that ate away at it over a long period of time. People experience the same thing. They will survive severe storms in their lives, but let themselves get eaten by the tiny bug of worry.

7. Look at the law of averages. What are the real odds of this worry happening? If it is a future worry, hardly any of them ever happen. Put it in the proper perspective. Sometimes the odds are nearly zero. If that is the case, it is foolish to give your thoughts much energy. If there is a possibility of the worry actually happening, a good question to ask yourself is, *"What is the worst thing that could happen if this does come about?"* What you will probably realize is that, even if the worst happens, it is usually not that bad. Our mind exaggerates the possibilities out of fear. So, even if it does happen, it usually is not devastating.

It is helpful to actually accept that the worst could happen. If you resolve to accept the worst, there is nothing left to worry about, and its significance diminishes. However, start taking steps to make sure the worst does not happen. Again, taking action —and any action will help — is the therapy. By doing so, you will not waste so much time in futile worry, and you will usually head off the worst case scenario.

8. Know when to walk away. When is enough, enough? Sometimes it is just not in our best interest to hang on to a particular issue. Usually, we do this to feel justified. We are trying not to be victimized or taken advantage of. Believe me, however, there are situations where it is best to cut your losses and move on. No more hanging on to a particular issue that is dragging you down, affecting your health, and preventing the flow of good things into your life. I think most of us have been there.

Years ago, I bought a house that was nothing but trouble from the beginning. The house needed a few custom alterations, but the builder and his staff were not easy to deal with, and I was having trouble getting things completed. It got to the point that I felt he was purposely being uncooperative for vindictive reasons. To make matters worse, he had an ongoing disagreement with the person from whom he bought the lot and I was caught in the middle. On top of that, the real estate company who listed the house did not have my best interests at heart.

I had the opportunity to get my deposit back and walk away, but I did not. I was within my rights to hold the builder to his word and get what I paid for, so I persisted. That was a big mistake. If I had it to do over again, I would have gotten out of the deal in the beginning and saved myself much unnecessary stress. The universe kept giving me hints, and I wouldn't listen. After I moved into the house I still was not happy, as problems continued on this hillside lot. The backyard was steep and the neighborhood was not as inviting as I had expected or hoped.

The point is that the time, energy, and money I expended were such a waste and held me back while I was entangled in the battle. For a small price in the beginning, I could have ended the situation quickly, with a minimal amount of drama. Sometimes you can win and still lose.

9. Do not saw sawdust. If you are worried about something in the past, you are wasting your time. It is done, move on. My suggestion is to get so busy with future goals, you do not have time to focus on the past. If you are beating yourself up over the past, stop. You did the best you could under those circumstances. It is not fair to judge yourself on the basis of today's circumstances. See the lesson clearly, and then learn from the past. Be aware you are using this past-focused worry to stop your future growth or justify your lack of future success. That thinking is for excuse-driven people, whining about why they're stuck or lost. That path is not for you. Take control like a winner. Get busy.

10. Live in the moment. Dale Carnegie talked about living in "day tight compartments" in his book, *How to Stop Worrying and Start Living*. Sometimes it can seem overwhelming when we look at our troubles. There are helpful steps to navigate your way out of the jungle, but to stay on course, break it down to one day at a time. That will keep you in the present and make everything possible. Carnegie reminds us to, *"Cross the bridge when you come to it, not before and not repeatedly."* When you think about doing something for thirty days, for example, that might seem difficult, even impossible. Think about doing it only today. Doesn't that feel lighter? Tomorrow you tell yourself the same thing, *"Just for today I will____."*

Not only does worry hold us back from our forward movement, it robs us of our peace and happiness. Again, I want to thank Brian Tracy for these ideas.

Here are six steps to help you live in peace and happiness every day:

1. Think and act cheerfully. Even if you do not feel like it, the more you do it the easier it will become. How does a cheerful, happy person stand, walk, sound, dress, and move? All of these things affect your emotional state. Some call this faking it until you make it, but I look at it all as a form of therapy. If you hunch over with your head down, how do you feel? If you talk in a whiney, monotone voice, how does that make you feel? You cannot separate the physical from the emotional. We are hardwired with one nervous system that innervates everything. Since we are connected with a common power source, doesn't it seem logical that it can affect anything (or everything)?

2. Do not try to get even or waste time thinking about people you do not like. There is a Navajo Proverb that sums it up: *"Thoughts are like arrows; once released they strike down their mark. Guard them well, or one day you may be your own victim."*

3. Express gratitude, but do not expect it. Give for the sake of giving with no strings attached. Jesus helped ten lepers in one day, and only one thanked him. Giving anonymously is powerful. Always look for ways to give. What you give does not always have to be material things. Compliments are always nice. Being kind and smiling is always welcome and, unfortunately, in too short of supply. Most people are starving for kindness. Try it, and see what it does for them. See what it does for you.

4. Be the best you. Many people are trying to be somebody else. It has been my observation that some have been playing certain roles so long, they are confused about whom they really are. Perhaps they have been shaped by other people's expectations of that which they should be, and they just assumed the role. People are happier when they are following their own paths and passions.

5. Focus on what you are grateful for. The Law of Attraction states that you become what you think about most of the time. Gratitude is a high vibrational form of love. Be grateful for what you have. Write more thank you notes! Be in a place of thankfulness for all your blessings, no matter how small. Focusing on what you have to be grateful for brings more gratitude into your life. Conversely, focusing on your problems or what you do not want will bring more of that as well.

6. Forget your worries by helping others. Simply put, happiness comes from helping others. By helping others, you help yourself. By being self-focused, you are directing energy inward. This can create dis-eases of the mind and body, including depression. A focus on serving others is a bigger vision to have. Directing your awareness outward will open doors to new, exciting paths that will help you discover who you really are and introduce you to the greatness within you, whether it is known to you or not. In the process, you are helping others achieve their potential. This is the ultimate win-win situation.

chapter FOUR

WATCH OUT FOR GOPHER HOLES

When I was fourteen years old, I was injured during the first week of freshman football practice. While running wind sprints during a nighttime practice on a poorly lit field, I stepped into a gopher hole. Obviously, we weren't practicing at AT&T Park. The shock of having the ground slip from beneath me was short-lived as the excruciating pain shot up my left leg and, with the very next step, I realized I couldn't put weight on it. Ever since then, I have had problems with it. I hobbled around for a year. No treatment was ever recommended or received, and, eventually, the pain subsided, but the injury remained.

I mention this story because of its symbolic importance to life. Life is full of gopher holes. Obviously, it behooves us to be aware they exist so we can avoid them if possible. If we should happen to step into one, it is best to resolve the situation as fast and effectively as we can. The sooner we resolve them the better, but later is definitely better than never.

Gopher holes can stop you in your tracks and prevent vibrant living. They can contribute to turning your physiological clock forward, rather than backward, becoming obstacles that halt your progression toward more youthfulness.

There are many types of gopher holes in life, including common holes that are avoidable. Some we create ourselves. For example, taking a risk by not using a seat belt or riding a bike without a helmet invites the possibility of self-induced gopher holes. I recently saw a man at a gas station lighting a cigarette as he filled up his car with gasoline. I had a hard time believing what I saw. This is a prime example of someone creating his own gopher hole. It makes sense to take certain preventative precautions.

Some gopher holes give us immediate feedback when we step into them. Others give us delayed results. Some gopher holes are obvious once we see them, and others are not. The ones we need to be particularly cautious of are those dressed up as something other than they really are, where the marketing differs from the reality. When it comes to ensuring a healthy future, it helps to have a basic understanding of which ingredients have the potential to help our brains and bodies and which have possible negative consequences.

The following are eight prevalent health gopher hole myths that people step into by the millions and put their future wellness at risk.

Myth: The lower your cholesterol is, the better off you are.

The low cholesterol myth has been perpetuated for quite a few years now. A basic understanding of how the body needs cholesterol should immediately alert you to the irrationality of this paradigm. Cholesterol is a necessary ingredient for health. It makes up a part of every cell membrane. It is a necessary ingredient for the body to make hormones. *The body needs cholesterol in order to function.* It is just ludicrous to look at it as some evil ingredient that must be eliminated.

Currently, there are three main erroneous approaches to the issue of cholesterol. The first myth is that the body produces too much of it. The second is that consuming too much cholesterol clogs arteries. The third myth is that the total cholesterol number needs to be lowered as much as possible.

The first myth, the idea that the body makes too much cholesterol, is interesting because there is no agreement about what is too much. Traditional medicine used to call a cholesterol level of 300 normal. When the first drugs were introduced to lower cholesterol, the normal range was lowered to 200 and, later, it was lowered even further.

If the diet is rich in cholesterol, the body will make less of it. Conversely, if the diet is devoid of it, the body will create more. The body self-regulates the amount in circulation. It is possible for the total cholesterol number to go very high, but I believe that this can point to either a delivery problem of getting it to where the body needs it or a problem in breaking down unused amounts.

Several areas can interfere with cholesterol utilization in the body. For example, the first step in using cholesterol for hormone synthesis is thyroid dependent. That means, your thyroid needs to be functioning optimally. If it is not, a thyroid problem could possibly affect a higher cholesterol number.

There are many other possible factors as to why the body is not utilizing cholesterol properly.

The second myth about cholesterol is the notion that consuming excessive amounts is the culprit in clogging arteries. There simply is not much supporting evidence. Most plaques are mostly calcium, not cholesterol, and the reason they are there has largely been ignored for years.

The homocysteine theory states that an injury to the arterial wall triggers a plaquing response by the body to patch the injury. Homocysteine is made during the breakdown of the amino acid methionine and should be neutralized very quickly. However, in the absence of certain nutrients, that doesn't happen. In particular, vitamin B6 and B12, folic acid, and magnesium are very important.

Homocysteine is a free radical that can damage artery walls. This information was never embraced because of the emphasis on recommending drugs to lower cholesterol. The only studies showing cholesterol was dangerous used oxidized (or rancid) cholesterol.

The third myth, which pushes to get cholesterol levels as low as possible, is a dangerous path to follow. Low cholesterol (I would consider less than 150 low) is associated with increased cancer risk, accidents, suicides, depression, and a drop in serotonin levels because the brain does not have enough good fuel — cholesterol — to support its basic functions. When the truth finally is widely accepted, I believe that low cholesterol will be shown to be more dangerous than high, and the treatments to lower cholesterol will be determined to be more dangerous than either low or high levels.

Using prescription drugs to lower cholesterol can affect muscle energy, so all types of muscle problems can result. The biggest danger is the possible weakening of the most important muscle — your heart. Because the statin drugs block the liver's ability to make coenzyme Q10, which is needed for muscle energy, the heart can weaken. A weakened heart condition is called congestive heart failure, which is on the rise dramatically in the U.S. as the number of statin prescriptions increases. Liver damage is another possible side effect of their use, which is just now starting to get attention in health literature.

The second component of current orthodox treatment consists of promoting a low cholesterol diet. This has to rank up there with the absolute worst medical advice ever given. Many of these no-cholesterol foods are very high in sugar and are loaded with trans fats. There is an undeniable correlation between sugar intake and cardiovascular disease. There is no good side to consuming trans fat. It is one of the worst things anybody can eat. A whole new fake food industry has been promoted in the name of health, when in fact it is the opposite of healthy. Plastic butter instead of the real thing and artificial eggs to make sure no one gets bad cholesterol are promoted as being "heart healthy."

Talk about a huge gopher hole. This myth should top the gopher hole Hall of Fame list.

Many times patients are surprised when they show me blood test results with the total cholesterol marked as being high, and I tell them not to worry about it. It is usually the least important finding on the whole test, and most of the time is not that high anyway. (I consider 180 to 210 or so just fine.) The current emphasis on high cholesterol is one of the biggest gopher holes out there today. The typical treatment plan is potentially harmful and diverts from real, more important factors. I can only conclude that plan is based more on marketing and sales than science and substance.

Myth: Aspirin is a health food.

Now, don't get me wrong, aspirin definitely has benefits that might be welcomed on a short-term basis. It seems hardly a week goes by that we do not hear of another newly discovered benefit of taking aspirin. It can relieve pain, and thin the blood, among other benefits, but to take it daily like a vitamin pill for health benefits needs to be examined a little closer.

Aspirin was discovered in 1899, so it has been around a while. While it is derived from salicin, a natural substance derived from white willow bark, aspirin is *not* natural. The active ingredient acetylsalicylic acid is synthetic.

Aspirin was used for seventy years before the mechanism of how it worked was understood. People just knew it worked. The anti-inflammatory effects come from its ability to block prostaglandin production. This brings pain relief, but there are also natural anti-inflammatory prostaglandins made by the body, and aspirin blocks those as well. That means it does not promote healing.

Probably the biggest medical reason for recommending aspirin today is for cardiovascular benefits. Evidence shows that aspirin may reduce the risk of a second non-fatal heart attack, but not fatal ones. It does not change the death rate, and people with high blood pressure do not get any benefit at all. One large study, in which 55,000 people participated, concluded aspirin could reduce the number of non-fatal heart attacks by 1% but would actually increase the risk of stroke, and there was no effect on mortality rates.

Possible side effects from regular aspirin use:

- Gastrointestinal bleeding and irritation.
- Increased risk of stroke.
- Macular degeneration with use of ten years or longer.
- Tripled death rate after angioplasty, when combined with ACE inhibitors.
- Acid reflux.
- Asthma attacks triggered 20 minutes to three hours after ingesting.
- Decreased kidney function. In a study of 100 elderly, 72 had decreased kidney function after two weeks on aspirin. By stopping the aspirin, kidney function improved.
- Liver problems, particularly if combined with alcohol.

- Ringing in the ears.
- Deafness.
- Pancreatic cancer.

In a study of 88,378 female nurses taking two or more aspirin a day for 20 years, 58% had an increase in pancreatic cancer. Those who consumed more than 14 tablets per week displayed an increase of 86%. This most likely has to do with the enzyme destroying capabilities of aspirin. Aspirin was actually one of the first preservatives used in the canning process to neutralize enzymes.

Again, I am not saying everybody should avoid using aspirin. There is a time and place for everything. However, when examined closely, I believe aspirin is more of a gopher hole than a healthy regular practice.

Myth: Heartburn and indigestion are caused by too much stomach acid.

Medicines for these conditions are some of the nation's biggest sellers. Consumers spend enormous amounts of money to alleviate this problem, based on a myth. The fact is that most people do not have enough stomach acid. *Stomach acid is required to digest food.* Attempts to eliminate stomach acid have harmful long-term consequences. (For a detailed description of how digestion works, see the first item "Stomach Pain" under natural remedies for 10 common health issues in Chapter 5.)

Most people do not have enough stomach acid, especially as they age. So, if there is discomfort right after eating, or a burning coming up the esophagus, what is going on? Usually it is an irritated stomach lining. The focus should be on healing the lining of the stomach rather than on eliminating acid and hindering digestion. By the way, undigested proteins can be very toxic to the body. They can trigger allergies, stress the kidneys, and increase the risk of colon cancer. Undigested proteins sitting in the intestines will putrefy just as they would in the trash. It has also been shown that some popular stomach medicines actually increase the populations of pathogenic bacteria in the stomach if they happen to be present.

Myth: High blood pressure is a disease. Once you have this disease you must be on medications the rest of your life.

This is a gopher hole that millions of Americans are stepping into. High blood pressure (HBP) is *not* a disease; it is a symptom of something being wrong in the pumps, pipes, or filters of the body. It is an effect, not a cause.

Using medication to force the blood pressure numbers down certainly has its place, but anytime you force a reaction in part of the body, there is a flip side to that coin. Also, in more than one-half of the patients it does not work. There is also not much evidence that taking medication prevents heart attacks at all. Probably the biggest benefit is to decrease stroke risk.

I remember years ago listening to a notable physician lecturing that more people have heart attacks on drug therapy than if they did nothing. Telling patients they have to stay on medication the rest of their lives is an admission the medication hasn't fixed the problem. Just changing the blood pressure numbers, or the numbers on a blood test, does not necessarily mean the problem has been solved. There are some benefits to taking medication, but you can still have an undetected dysfunction taking place that needs more help to alleviate the stress the body is experiencing.

A common issue found along with high blood pressure is a circulatory problem. If something is clogging the arteries it will cause the blood pressure to go up. Kidney stress is very common, particularly with high systolic pressure (the top number) that stays high laying or standing. High blood sugar can trigger high blood pressure because blood sugar can cause the arteries to constrict. Stress, which affects blood sugar, also causes constriction of vessels.

The garden hose analogy works here. You can increase water pressure two ways. You can turn the faucet on higher to pump more water through the hose, or tighten the nozzle and increase the resistance to the outflow. If you think of your arteries as the hose, that is exactly what happens. High blood pressure means an increase in internal resistance or pressure. Anything that causes this will have an effect.

In my experience, many people with high blood pressure are wound up pretty tight. They are not calm or at peace. They often have their guard up and frequently try to control their environment. Along with the physical approaches, like yoga, meditation, and slow walking meditation, other therapies that help in dealing with life can be crucial for success. There is no magic prescription pill that will accomplish this.

Myth: Vaccinations keep you healthy and increase your immunity.

Every year there is a massive campaign to vaccinate people for the flu, and the pressure to have your children vaccinated is never ending. I won't debate the efficacy of the vaccines (and it *is* debatable), but will rather make the point that vaccines are a massive gopher hole, and in my opinion, in almost all cases the benefits are not worth the risks. Vaccines are toxic, and you are better off with non-toxic, natural approaches whenever possible. The heavy metals and preservatives found in vaccines are *not* health-producing. Quite the contrary.

What about the benefits of immunity? Vaccines do produce an immune response, but any toxic or infectious agent will do that. This artificially triggered response is to man-made pathogens and is not the same as building immunity or a memory of how to defend against certain diseases. Natural immunity is the only true immunity, and it happens after being exposed to the illness. With vaccines, you are creating antibodies to an artificial version produced in a lab, rather than a naturally occurring illness.

A final comment about the effectiveness of the shots is this: American children are the most vaccinated children in the world. If vaccines equaled health, they should be the healthiest. They are not. It has been my observation over the years that the healthiest children I have seen in my practice did not receive vaccinations. They do not experience the chronic ear infections, asthma, or unexplained high fevers. There also is a marked difference in their disposition.

Once vaccines have been introduced, I believe that a number of behavior problems can manifest because the child simply does not feel well. It is not unusual for children to feel poorly immediately after vaccinations. They will become irritable, clingy, or have a fever. There may also be long-term effects, such as chronic ear infections, which can begin immediately. This topic fits into the gopher hole category because parents and consumers are not given the whole story: that the benefits of vaccinations are overstated, risks are understated, and their use is perpetuated by fear and propaganda. I will admit that I am biased on this subject because my oldest son actually had a severe reaction to a vaccination as a child. In those days, pediatricians had posters hanging in their offices that said only one child in two hundred and fifty thousand had an adverse reaction to vaccinations. I found out later that, at that time, there had *never* been a safety study done. So where did that number come from? Why were there posters to reassure parents?

Myth: If a food is marketed as healthy, it is.

Talk about a health gopher hole. There are no limits to the depths some companies will go to sell their products. The real kicker here is that many get help from certain health, medical, and government agencies.

It was revealed a couple of years ago that a cereal product bearing the logo of an organization that promotes heart health, actually paid for the rights to use the logo. Can you believe that? The healthy agency's logo was for sale. It had nothing to do with the quality of the product in the box. Millions of people saw that logo and assumed it was a healthy product.

It is not safe to assume these days. Assuming creates gopher holes. Some sources have proven to be more truthful than others. However, you must educate yourself about what is or is not healthy, what are credible sources of information, and of whom you need to be particularly wary.

With all of the contradictory information out there, how do you know what to believe? The safest answer is to not believe any of it, and instead do your own research. If an organization has a past history of being deceitful and untruthful time after time, why waste your time and energy focusing on what they have to say? Chances are they are once again trying to sway public opinion to fit their agenda rather than tell you the truth. They do not deserve your attention.

Many of these organizations are in positions of authority and power. Your welfare is not at the top of their priority list. This goes for certain private as well as government groups. For example, many Americans have forgotten (or never knew) that smoking was once promoted as healthy. There actually were financial ties between organizations to promote this perception. The government also told people that above-ground nuclear testing was not harmful, and that any radiation exposure was actually beneficial. The list goes on and on. I think my point is clear.

Some large organizations fund groups to discredit those who disagree with them. They target critics of fast food, alcohol, mercury-laden fish, and any drugs. They will promote junk foods as healthy, and their critics as kooks. For example, Tufts University School of Nutrition qualified a cereal that is 41% sugar, loaded with hydrogenated fats and artificial colors for its "Smart Choices" label. The dean of a nationally recognized school defended sugar in children's foods as a good thing so children will eat more of it. A popular baby formula was recently recalled because some foreign material was found in it. The *Natural News* newsletter reported that the recall missed a very important issue: The formula had a total of 52% sugar content. I do not believe this gives children a great start to life.

There is no nutrition in refined sugar. In fact, it robs nutrients from the body, making it a negative food. Either these people are so nutritionally ignorant it boggles the mind they are considered experts, or they are just reciting what they are told to say by their employers or sponsor, and they really do not care about sounding competent. The tragedy is we have adult individuals and certain corporations selling out our children. Shouldn't we be protecting our children?

Myth: Drugs create health.

It is no wonder we have such a drug problem in the U.S. Talk about mixed messages. With many commercials on television being drug ads and people watching hours of it daily, the programming is strong and constant. The American government has a strong bias toward drugs, and they use (or misuse) their authority against non-drug therapies.

The official stance of the FDA is that only drugs can change physiology. I wonder what they think food does? 90% of drug addicts in the U.S. are addicted to legal drugs. With all the advertising and emphasis on drugs for every type of ailment, I expect that number to go up. Drugs are used to treat disease, but they cannot create or maintain health. Drugs can save lives, and that certainly is a good thing.

However, all drugs have side effects. The unintentional injury and deaths from poisoning is on the rise, and most are from prescription drugs. In 2008, the Poison Control Center stated that over 100,000 deaths were due to pre-scription drugs. That same year, there were no deaths from natural supplements. In addition, it has been reported that every year 700,000 emergency room visits are attributed to side effects of legal drugs, compared to 10,000 visits from those of illegal drugs. Drugs are drugs, and the only real difference between the legal and illegal ones is how they are given and who is making the profit.

Warning people about the dangers of illegal drugs on one hand, and then telling them they need to be on multiple legal drugs on the other, is the height of malicious hypno-tism. Unfortunately, the number of celebrity deaths at the hands of legal drug abuse has done little to change the tide of the land. The drug push is successful. In one ten-year period (1997–2007), the number of prescriptions rose by 72%. In 2004 alone there were four billion prescriptions written. We are the most medicated country in the world. If legal drugs resulted in an increase in health and wellness we should be the healthiest country.

The truth is however, that the U.S. is *not* the healthiest. It ranks dead last in health statistics in the industrialized world and pays more for these drugs in the U.S. than anywhere else. Drugs from outside of the country are publicized as potentially dangerous, but the fact is, the same drug can be purchased in another country like Mexico for considerably less than in the U.S. What the media does not say is that many high-priced U.S. drugs are actually made in Puerto Rico where it is much cheaper to produce them.

It is apparent that drugs do not equal health. Emergency medicine can be seen separately as a short-term approach to get patients stabilized. However, long-term healthcare using a variety of drugs, an average of 13 drugs per year for every American over age 65, is a gopher hole.

Myth: Antibiotics are the best way to treat sinus and ear infections.

This is a gopher hole because antibiotics should be used to treat bacterial infections only, and most sinus and ear infections are not bacterial infections. This is worth mentioning since over 20% of antibiotic prescriptions in the U.S. are for sinus infections. Chronic sinus infections are usually a symptom of a fungal problem. Even the Mayo

Clinic said most (over 90%) of sinus infections were positive for fungus, not bacteria. That being the case, antibiotics would *not* be an effective treatment, and they could actually make the problem worse since they promote yeast and fungal growth. Yes, symptoms do change sometimes after antibiotics are taken, but relief is usually only for a limited time and the infection often comes raging back.

The sinuses are actually an overflow valve for the body. They are used as a route for elimination. A sinus infection can mean that the body is not eliminating through normal channels properly. For example, many sinus problems are actually related to lung issues, and that is where therapy should often be focused in order to resolve the sinus infection.

Ear infections are often similarly misdiagnosed. Most chronic childhood ear infections have been shown not to be infections. In these cases the ears are not the problem, but a symptom of another problem. Just because the inner ear hurts and the ear drum is red does not mean it is infected. If it is not and antibiotics are given, the problem usually comes back with a vengeance in short order. Children at times will display lymphatic congestion if the kidneys need help with their drainage function. If the body can't eliminate properly, there is a backup in the lymphatic system. Mucus is a byproduct created from inflammation and it builds up behind the ears. One study concluded there was not a bacterial infection present in over 60% of the cases. With no bacterial infection present, antibiotics are not the appropriate treatment, and will not alleviate the congestion on a long term basis.

There has even been little-publicized but credible medical research saying that antibiotics were not the best treatment for chronic inner ear problems. However, I have not seen much change over the past 20 years in how these problems are treated.

I encourage people to look around and become more aware. How well does treating these problems with antibiotics really work? Once children start the antibiotic merry-go-round, their health can suffer in a number of ways. Antibiotics suppress the immune system. They also can cause intestinal problems like diarrhea and pain, and it is common for children to not be as healthy as they were before taking them. There is a time and place for everything, and antibiotics do have beneficial uses. However, regarding sinus and ear problems, antibiotic use is a big gopher hole that often becomes part of a bigger problem, instead of a solution.

The best scenario is to avoid gopher holes altogether, but that is not always realistic. Once a gopher hole has been stepped in, it is important to take corrective action quickly. For example, if there were a physical injury (as in the football injury I mentioned at the beginning of the chapter), it is best to find an expert in treating such injuries like a chiropractor, physical therapist, a good body worker, or massage therapist, who can administer a variety of treatments such as myofascial release, **Quantum Neurology**® (which balances the nervous system using light therapy), Bowen therapy, **Rolfing**®, or cranial sacral therapy as soon as possible.

The sooner the better is my motto. If I can get a whip-lash patient in my office the day of the accident, often we can erase the damage very quickly and the consequences experienced are mild to none. It is frequently possible to either fix the problem or minimize the long-term effects. Literally resetting the nervous system and making specific adjustments to the body and brain can put the body back into a pre-accident state, almost like it never happened.

chapter FIVE

NATURE'S PHARMACY

Our creator blessed us with marvelous natural medicines for health and healing. What was not supplied, however, was a user's manual for these remedies and how beneficial they are. We are left to fend for ourselves when learning about and applying natural remedies.

I have often felt envious of people born into situations that benefited their knowledge base in this area. I have a friend who was born in Mexico whose grandmother was an herbalist. Whatever was ailing the children, she knew the remedy. I was the beneficiary of her knowledge once when I burned my arm. I put aloe vera gel from a bottle on it. It brought some relief but still looked bad.

My friend Martina informed me that, according to her grandmother, what I needed was not from a bottle, but the actual plant. She sliced a piece of an aloe vera leaf and taped it over the burn. The improvement in one day was amazing. I was informed that the "sticky stuff" from the plant was important and it did not come from a bottle.

Did she know what the sticky stuff was called? No. I am sure her grandmother did not know either. I did not care; it worked great. Many grandmothers used to be herbalists and healers. This is no longer the case as this wisdom is not being passed down any more. That fact, along with the increasing censorship regarding non-pharmaceutical remedies, is making it much more difficult to access valuable information.

The natural medicine paradigm differs from the medical paradigm in a number of ways. Both have value but are different in their core concepts and philosophies. I believe it is important to discuss the differences, because if people want to try the natural approach but their thoughts and expectations are along the orthodox path in most cases they will not be satisfied with the outcome.

It is worth noting that before World War II there were more homeopathic doctors and herbalists in the United States than there were pharmaceutically oriented physicians. During the war there was a surge in chemical warfare research and development, which was the impetus for drug development and marketing of these new "medicines." There followed a successful campaign to eliminate much of the natural practitioner population by using legislation, the popular press, and other heavy handed techniques.

Today, however, there is an ever increasing interest in natural medicine. One of the biggest differences is the main focus of each particular discipline. Medicine emphasizes finding a disease and then treating that disease using drugs or surgery in most cases, while natural medicine emphasizes restoring balance and function.

Increasing numbers of people are realizing they want more from health care than just disease diagnosis. People are becoming aware that what they eat and drink, and how they think and move, are extremely important to their overall health picture. There are major limitations to disease diagnosis being the primary objective. For one, there is very little, if anything, done for prevention. Waiting until the late stages of ill health to implement treatment is expensive, especially when compared to the results. The concept of making healthy changes in one's lifestyle to prevent disease later is rarely a consideration. This is changing somewhat, and there are some outstanding medical doctors doing great work in preventative health care, but these doctors are the exception, not the rule.

Another limitation of traditional medicine is the emphasis on symptomatic relief, rather than a comprehensive analysis of what is causing the problem. It is, for the most part, a segmentally oriented system. A tumor, for example, is viewed as the problem, rather than an effect of what is causing the tumor to form. If someone is fatigued, they may be given an antidepressant rather than look for the cause of the fatigue.

A major drawback to traditional medicine is that if no disease is found it is assumed there are no real problems to be concerned with. The concept of one being either healthy or having a disease is simply not realistic. Most people have signs and symptoms that can be precursors to a disease later on if not dealt with appropriately. This happens to the majority of patients who, in my opinion, seldom get the treatment and advice needed.

A disease does not develop overnight. It is a process of stress and degeneration that usually goes on for some time. To ignore the warning signs until the late stages of ill health is not the most beneficial approach. The natural approach does not ignore signs and symptoms, but rather views them as warnings of an imbalance. It does not assume the symptoms are where the problem is. The interconnectedness of all the body's symptoms is appreciated.

Disease care is *not* health care, and it is time we get honest about what is, and is not, being delivered. As I mentioned previously, both have their place, but the role of natural health care should be the main source of health care, except in cases of trauma, and not put at the back of the bus and called "alternative." There is nothing alternative about it.

Why use natural remedies when we have all these pharmaceutical medicines available today? For one, natural remedies are safer. Drugs can have powerful affects and side effects. Due to the popular press and television ads many people are more afraid of natural remedies than drugs and surgery. We are truly living in upside down times.

There is a tremendous amount of corporate influence at play here. Natural remedies are cheaper. But, because insurance will not cover the cost in most cases, it has the appearance of being more expensive. Nothing could be further from the truth. Not everybody agrees with this because health insurance covers the prescription drugs while natural remedies are often purchased out-of-pocket. While we may not have to pay directly, somebody certainly is paying for these drugs and some prescriptions are extremely expensive. The appearance of medicine being paid for does not make it free. Current Medicare and traditional insurance practices are contributing to bankrupting the country. There are simply not enough doctors and not enough money to pay for a "disease care" system.

Natural remedies are more effective in many cases. Exceptions to this are emergency medicine and pain relievers. But, for health issues and chronic degenerative diseases, there are very effective natural solutions. When I hear people in the media and so-called health experts talk about how worthless the natural ways are, I always wonder, *"If it were so ineffective, why would they go to these great lengths using lies, phony studies, censorship, and many other unethical tactics to discredit it?"* If natural remedies did not work, nobody would want them, but that is not the case. It reminds me of something Einstein said when a hundred scientists colluded to write a book on why he was wrong. His response was, *"If I was really wrong, only one would be needed."*

My intention is not to downplay the benefits of orthodox medicine, but to point out that benefits of natural medicine are greater than most people realize. My two-fold goal is not to give specific advice, but to increase awareness and give an overview of natural treatments for common ailments. Drugs have their place, particularly in treating disease; however, they do not create balance in the body or maintain good health. Natural remedies, on the other hand, do have these abilities if used appropriately.

The following are some of my favorite remedies for common conditions from which people suffer today. Obviously, this information is just that, information, and is not intended to diagnose or be used as specific medical advice. If you are being treated for a condition by your doctor, do not make any changes without consulting him or her first.

Here are natural remedies for 10 common health issues:

Stomach pain

The enormous dollar volume spent on over-the-counter medicines, such as antacids, gastric reflux remedies, constipation, and diarrhea medicines to obtain relief indicate that indigestion is a major problem in our country. Many indigestion relief medicines are based on the model that there is too much stomach acid, and that this excessive acid is causing the discomfort. This is an erroneous assumption, as most people experience the opposite problem, particularly as they age, and do not have *enough* stomach acid.

A little basic physiology is in order here. The digestive enzyme pepsin, not acid, digests protein in the stomach. After a meal, it takes about 45 minutes for enough acid to accumulate in the stomach to drop the pH low enough to liberate the enzyme pepsin from pepsinogen. If there is not enough acid, then pepsin will not be present and digestion will suffer. This question always comes up, *"Don't doctors know this?"* My answer is that the majority do not because, again, most medical education focuses on disease and the treatment of the disease, not on function.

Then what causes the discomfort? Burning and pain in the stomach immediately after eating (remember, there is no acid in the stomach at this time) is often diagnosed as gastric reflux, but is usually from an irritated stomach lining. It is also possible that ulcers are present or are starting to form.

What needs to happen is healing of the gastric lining. Some effective remedies can usually bring about relief in a very short period of time. Slippery elm, deglycyrrhizinated licorice (DGL), marshmallow, an ounce or two of fresh, uncooked cabbage juice, and the amino acid L-glutamine can also be helpful. If there is a bacterial infection (like H. pylori), natural or pharmaceutical antibiotics would need to be employed. A berberine remedy or grapefruit seed extract can be added to get the infection under control.

One of the simplest, cheapest and most important remedies for dyspepsia, or stomach pain, is water. According to the book, *Your Body's Many Cries for Water* by Fereydoon Batamanghelidj, chronic dehydration is the underlying cause of most dyspepsia. When the body is dehydrated, the lining of the stomach actually shrinks in thickness making the stomach more prone to irritation. Irritation could also mean a need for more sodium, since sodium is what holds on to water in the body. This is one connection between stress and ulcers. Under constant stress the body loses sodium in the urine and there is more sodium in the stomach than anywhere else. So, stress causes sodium to be lost, which means the body does not hold on to water. This leads to dehydration and a shrinking of the gastric lining, which leads to stomach irritation, pain, and possibly gastric reflux or ulcers over time. The many millions of dollars people are spending on medicines do not fix any of this, and in fact, further interfere with the digestive process. I will elaborate on this topic in the next chapter.

Pain and inflammation

Pain medications are also some of the top sellers. For quick pain relief, drugs can be very effective. However, taking these medicines long-term can have side effects. I feel the recommendation to take an aspirin a day is ill-advised in most cases. Non-steroidal anti-inflammatory drugs also can affect the gut and the kidneys. Acetaminophen is very toxic to the liver. One of its effects is to deplete glutathione, which is very important for liver function. Taking a bottle of acetaminophen can kill you, so in some other countries it is sold in smaller packages to prevent death by over-dosing.

Natural anti-inflammatories can lessen the need for so many drugs and, for long-term use, they are much kinder to the body. Some drugs can block the body's natural anti-inflammatory response, so these do not promote healing.

Bromelain is a proteolytic enzyme that does a great job of keeping inflammation in check and also helps the body repair in the case of an injury. Other enzymes can be potent anti-inflammatories. For example, when taken in between meals, amylase can help skin problems and rashes where there is heat and redness. Insect bites, poison oak, and allergic reactions can be helped with amylase. The inflammatory response of redness is the clue to use amylase. It is also beneficial in easing muscle soreness and joint stiffness. When taken in between meals lipase can help with the inflammatory response of swelling and lymphatic congestion.

Essential fatty acids and oils like coconut, fish, and krill have anti-inflammatory characteristics. Wheat germ oil is also good against intestinal inflammation.

Many herbs are also powerful anti-inflammatories. Yucca is a great Southwestern herbal anti-inflammatory. It can be used for anything from swollen prostates to painful knees. I have seen it be particularly effective for osteoarthritis pain. Celery is also a good anti-inflammatory. It can help osteoarthritis, gout, psoriasis, and shingles. Celery is a great source of sodium, which most people with arthritis need. There are others, like devil's claw and boswellia, but two of my favorite remedies are ginger and turmeric.

If I could have only two items in the medicine cabinet, they would be the spices ginger and turmeric. They are both so valuable in treating such a wide variety of ailments that many people could drastically reduce their dependency on toxic, synthetic drugs by implementing these two gems. Over the years, I have found that many are slow to accept remedies that are simple, inexpensive, and readily available. The question that arises from time to time is, "*Are they proven to work?*" The answer is, "*Yes, they are.*" Natural remedies have been used effectively for centuries by civilizations who appreciated their value, and many studies have been done proving their efficacy.

Ginger has been called the natural aspirin, because it offers many of the benefits of aspirin, such as thinning the blood and pain relief, without side effects, like gastrointestinal bleeding and kidney stress. Ginger has the additional advantage of being an herbal antibiotic against bacterial pathogens like E. coli and Salmonella.

Here are more medicinal uses of ginger:

- Cold and flu remedy
- Expectorant and antihistamine
- Aids upper respiratory infections
- Reduces inflammation and fevers
- Topical treatment for burns and blisters
- Relieves arthritis joint pain
- Reduces nausea
- Aids digestion
- Helps headaches

Turmeric is almost as versatile. Curcumin is the active ingredient that appears to supply most of the health benefits, of which there are many.

Here is a partial list of turmeric's benefits:

- Protects the liver and gall bladder from damage by chemicals and toxins they deal with daily.
- Functions as an anti-inflammatory. With turmeric, arthritis pain can be reduced without suppressing the body's ability to make its own anti-inflammatory substances and create new cells. Turmeric has been proven to be even more effective for pain and stiffness than many big-selling drugs.
- Increases antioxidants. Glutathione, along with anthocyanins (found in berries), have been shown to normalize cancer cells in German research. Turmeric ingestion helps produce more glutathione.
- Suppresses amyloid plaques that cause Al-

zheimer's disease. Inflammation and free radical damage appear to cause most dementia and nerve dysfunction that are epidemic today. Turmeric has been shown to reduce this inflammation and protect the brain.

- Shown to protect organs from chemotherapy toxicity. It also helps anti-cancer drugs work better.

Both ginger and turmeric have such a wide variety of possible uses, are very safe to use, and have withstood the test of time. They would be a valuable addition to any medicine cabinet.

Natural antibiotics

Beyond ginger and turmeric, several more herbs have antibiotic abilities. Garlic has been shown to be very effective against intestinal bacteria. Since intestinal problems are on the rise, garlic is so readily available, and antibiotics are less effective than they used to be, the timing is right for people to know what garlic can do. Garlic is also an excellent cold and flu remedy. It is best taken at the first sign of illness. It also has anti-yeast and anti-fungal benefits and is a great remedy for chronic sinus infections.

Goldenseal is one of the better known herbal antibiotics. Goldenseal seems to work best for acute infections and inflammation of the gastrointestinal tract. It can also be used topically for skin infections. It is great for cleansing the blood, too. The root is the strongest part of the herb and has anti-inflammatory properties.

Echinacea, sage, grapefruit seed extract and usnea are also very effective natural antibiotics. Echinacea is helpful against infections like strep throat. It is often combined with other herbs like goldenseal. Sage is particularly useful against gastrointestinal infections, as well as throat and upper respiratory infections. Grapefruit seed extract is one of the more powerful natural remedies. It has strong antibiotic properties, but also works as an anti-yeast and anti-fungal. Usnea is one of the stronger remedies. It also has anti-fungal properties and is effective against several strains of bacteria. It has been shown to be particularly effective against lung infections (like tuberculosis). Usnea is also good for skin infections, wounds, and abscesses.

Juniper and uva ursi help combat urinary tract infections. D-mannose and dried herbal cranberry are widely used. Cranberry prevents the bacteria from adhering to the lining of the urinary tract, and d-mannose treats the infection itself. I prefer the herbal form of cranberry to the juice, which has a high fructose content that feeds the bacteria.

Boneset helps with flues where fever and chills are present. It can also be very beneficial for upper respiratory infections that are "full blown."

Other herbs with antibiotic characteristics include aloe, acacia, eucalyptus, barberry, and Oregon grape root. With antibiotic resistance growing rapidly, it is time we re-learned what used to be commonly known.

If the illness is viral in nature, there are several beneficial herbs: elderberry, isatis, andrographis, osha root, and astragalus. Several years ago in Beijing, China, there was an outbreak of viral encephalitis and the police were dispensing isatis from large drums to people on the streets. It worked to stop the epidemic. The isatis I like is a tincture from Dragon River Herbals in New Mexico. They also carry most of the herbal remedies I mentioned here.

Headaches

This is such a common complaint it is worthy of noting. A headache can definitely ruin the day. I am always amazed at how long some people have struggled with this problem. It is not unusual for patients to tell me they have been dealing with their headaches for ten or fifteen years.

In my years of treating headaches, I have observed some common themes. In my opinion, these are the causes of most non-traumatically induced headaches:

Stress

Many people are on overload much of the time.

When stress wins over our ability to handle it, blood vessels constrict, muscles contract, then the vessels dilate. When they dilate, they stretch nerve fibers that wrap around them, and a headache is the result. Many people are working at jobs they dislike and are living in less than ideal environments. Supporting the adrenal glands and some stress reduction strategies are needed. To this end, ashwagandha has a calming effect on moods. 5 hydroxytryptophan (5-HTP) also has a calming effect. GABA can be used if recurrent negative thoughts are at the source of the stress; it is an inhibitory neurotransmitter which puts the brakes on unwanted thoughts. Many people partake in stress-relieving habits that further contribute to their headaches. Too much alcohol, caffeine, chocolate, or sugar, are common culprits.

Ileocecal valve problems

The ileocecal valve (ICV) is between the small and large intestine. It is very susceptible to pH changes and is easily disturbed by pathogenic organisms and when exposed to food allergens. When it malfunctions, it may allow seepage of waste material that should be moving out, back into the small intestine. This is like a sewer line leaking into your kitchen. This creates an irritation that affects the nerve supply to the intestines, which then reflexes to the neck, and can trigger a headache. Many times there will be a marked decrease in head rotation to the right with an ICV problem. Digestive enzymes taken with meals, and possibly the elimination of pathogens, may be necessary. To soothe the ICV, fat-soluble chlorophyll does a nice job, as water-soluble does not reach that far down in the intestines. Many times the addition of a good probiotic will resolve these headaches. There will usually be a weak iliacus muscle when muscle testing the right side as well. The iliacus muscle tests weak because the same nerve that enervates the lower right quadrant of the intestines also enervates the ilacus muscle, which is also discussed under the back pain section below.

Blood sugar imbalances

If the blood sugar drops too low, it can trigger a stress response by forcing the adrenal glands to bring it back up. Again, vessels constrict and muscles contract. These headaches can be severe. Paying attention to eating habits is necessary here. Keeping the sugar and refined carbohydrates out of the diet, eating regular meals, increasing water, and taking appropriate supplements are key. Sometimes chromium, magnesium, vitamin B1, or digestive enzymes are needed to normalize blood sugar. Herbs like gymnema sylvestre are also helpful. Pancreatic enzymes and plant enzymes can be beneficial as well. Besides eating the wrong foods, skipping meals can also be a headache trigger for some, as is prolonged work without breaks.

Migraines

It is my experience that migraines almost always include liver stress as part of the problem. Now, the cause of that liver stress may be different with different people. Common stresses include a toxic colon, since the primary job of the liver is to detox the colon, a food allergy, nutritional deficiency, or hormonal fluctuations. Red wine, certain cheeses, and bananas are common villains. Riboflavin and magnesium can be useful in aborting or turning down the volume of a migraine. Riboflavin usually needs to be taken in the range of 200 to 400 mg at a time.

Back pain

The majority of Americans will experience back pain at some point in their lives. The treatments that are most commonly employed are not very successful for long-term solutions. Some do provide temporary, symptomatic relief. One study on all back treatments came to the conclusion they are all ineffective, from back surgery to more conservative treatments. Months later everyone treated was in nearly the same condition. In fact, treatments were rated by which ones hurt the patient the least, not by what helped people the most. In one study, yoga and Applied

Kinesiology were the only two treatments that did not make anyone worse. Back surgery fails so often it has its own insurance code. My contention is that an erroneous model is used by most treatments, thus failure is the only reasonable outcome. The medical model most widely used places the location of the pain as the cause of the problem. It is not the cause, but rather an effect. Pain-relieving drugs will not fix the problem. A natural approach can and will, except in a small percentage of the cases, where surgery is necessary.

In my clinical experience, there are three common causes of back pain:

The intestinal connection

An imbalance in the ecological system of the intestines, particularly when it affects the ileocecal valve, can cause low back pain. In my experience, this is the most common cause of low back disc problems. The imbalance in the intestines will irritate the nerve supply back to the spine and affect the muscles innervated by that same nerve. The iliacus, which is a broad pelvic stabilizing muscle, neurologically weakens and allows for pelvic rotation. The nerve innervation arises from the first lumbar vertebrae, but the pelvic rotation will put sheer pressure on the lower vertebrae. The pain is usually at the L-5, S-1 nerve roots. The pelvic rotation squeezes the disc, much like pinching one end of a balloon. Until the stimulus for the rotation is resolved, the problem will persist.

The actual cause for the intestinal issue can be different with individual patients. Too much unfriendly bacteria, parasites, yeast, and constipation are common problems that need attention. Once the stimulus is corrected and the pelvic rotation is no longer there, therapies applied to the back will have a greater result. Berberine, oregano, grapefruit seed extract, garlic, artemesia annua, black walnut, and probiotics are all natural remedies I use on a regular basis. Proteolytic enzymes help reduce the swelling and pain in the back and promote repair. When taken as a remedy for inflammation, it is important that the enzymes be consumed in between meals for maximum benefit. If taken with food, they work on digestion. Approaching this type of back pain from this model brings rapid positive results, far beyond what the textbooks say is possible.

Kidney stress
Kidney stress can cause back pain a couple of ways. The kidneys themselves can hurt and since they are located in the back that is where you feel it. Usually this pain will be just below the posterior ribs. Another way the kidneys cause pain is the muscle-organ

relationship. The kidneys share the same nerve supply as the quadratus lumborum muscles, which extend from the bottom of the ribs in the back down to the pelvis. These muscles are involved because the nerve irritation causes the muscles to spasm, and there will be stiffness and pain, usually at the muscle attachments. This pain can be very sharp and will usually be triggered by rotation movements. This pain can be debilitating and severely restrict what movement is possible.

To treat this type of back pain, the source (the kidneys) must be treated. Alfalfa is a wonderful herb for the kidneys, as are mullein, parsley, American ginseng and several others. Proteolytic enzymes can also be helpful to the kidneys, particularly when the pollen count is high. Pollens that are not broken down by the body can stress the kidneys. It is also important to stay well-hydrated and eliminate certain foods. Milk and milk products are common offenders. I have seen long-term back sufferers get tremendous relief just by eliminating milk from their diet. Cold drinks and sugar should be dropped. Foods that are good for the kidneys include asparagus, spinach, parsley, adzuki beans, and adzuki bean tea is excellent. Mix two tablespoons of beans and two quarts of water, boil down to one quart and sip as tea. This tea is one of the most effective treatments for strengthening the kidneys I have witnessed over the years.

Nervous system imbalance

The autonomic nervous system is composed of the sympathetic and parasympathetic components. An imbalance in this system, where either component has become predominate, can cause lower back pain. They should both be in equal balance.

Here is what happens. Acidic tissues can cause heat, inflammation, and pain. People can experience pain when the sympathetic nervous system is dominant because they tend to be acidic. The sympathetic nervous system is comprised of the spinal nerves. A stress response is a sympathetic nerve response. The adrenal glands are our stress glands. The adrenal glands might be pumping out cortisol like crazy. The muscle-organ correlation to the adrenals is the Sartorius muscle, which is a pelvic stabilizer, as well as a medial knee muscle. That is why under stress, which happens a lot with athletes, knee injuries are common. On the side of Sartorius weakness, the sacroiliac joint will become unstable, and this alone can cause pain. There can be more causes of pain, however. When the sacroiliac joint, (also called the SI joint) becomes unstable, the lower lumbar vertebrae will have a tendency to rotate to compensate. The third lumbar will usually become a problem, as that is the nerve source to the Sartorius; but with the SI issue, the fifth lumbar will usually subluxate, and that usually causes the most pain.

To stop this pattern, the person needs to calm their nervous system, cool off the body with fresh fruits, more green foods, and eliminate heat-producing foods like caffeine, sugar and alcoholic beverages, and the stress response must be dealt with. B vitamins, choline, and regular exposure to blue light may be very useful. American ginseng, osha, and ashwagandha are worthy of consideration. Alkalizing the system can be useful as well. Consuming green foods and lemon water, and eliminating red meat, sugar, and caffeine are all good choices. High doses of calcium are contraindicated in this case, but potassium and magnesium supplementation would be recommended.

With a parasympathetic imbalance, back pain is also a possibility, but the cause is different. The parasympathetic nervous system is the nerves that arise from the sacrum and the cranium. Because the sacrum makes up part of the SI joints, it is common to see stress and weakness in those joints, often bilaterally. When the SI joints weaken, the gluteus maximus muscles will also weaken. These are the big muscles in your hind end. They are major work horses. They are needed for lifting and getting up from a seated position. People who must use their arms to help themselves up, or lean on shopping carts in the grocery store for back support, usually have this weakness. The inguinal ligament on the front side of the body (in the groin line) will tighten to compensate for the weakness on the back side. Smaller muscles will now have to do more of the work they are not designed to do, and this can lead to back pain.

As time goes on, the inguinal ligament tightness can affect the nerves innervating the quadriceps muscles in the thighs. As they become weaker, it becomes more difficult to walk up stairs and lift the legs up. This can also affect the hips and knees. This person would benefit from more meat and higher doses of calcium and vitamin D. Oat straw and Shiitake mushroom are two good supplements. If you are also prone to anxiety and panic attacks, kava kava is worth considering for these episodes. There may also be protein metabolism issues, which are common with this imbalance, that need to be dealt with.

To assist in healing, exercises that contract the gluteus maximus muscles are beneficial. For example, lying prone with one leg bent, lift it toward the ceiling slowly and carefully.

You can also do this standing. The point is to bring one leg to extension, preferably with the knee bent. You can also contract and relax the gluteus maximus muscles, also called glute squeezes. Start activating these muscles, as if you were holding something with them, by contracting, holding for a few seconds, relaxing them, and repeating.

Immune boosters

Keeping the immune system strong is important to be able to defend against illness, and there are several excellent herbal remedies that help achieve this goal. One of the best is astragalus. Astragalus is particularly effective in the early stages of an infection. It helps with general immunity, boosting the spleen's functioning. It has antiviral properties and is generally one of the better remedies for a flu or cold. Shiitake mushroom also boosts general immunity to fend off both viruses and bacteria. Siberian ginseng is an effective immune enhancer for people who are depleted and have exhausted immune systems. Some females and people over forty may find it too stimulatory, in which case licorice or American ginseng may be a better choice.

Maitake mushroom is excellent for supporting specific immunity, particularly related to the thymus gland. The thymus produces natural killer cells, which are so important in dealing with infection and abnormal cells in the body. Maitake is one of my favorites for aiding thymus function. Reishi is another great mushroom for the immune system. Combining the mushrooms together can be extremely powerful to aid healing.

Specific vitamins also help immunity, particularly vitamins C and A. Vitamin C has antibacterial as well as antiviral properties. In acute stages of infection, higher dosages can be beneficial (3,000 to 6,000 mg per day). I do not recommend dosages this high on an ongoing basis. Vitamin A is particularly effective with viral infections. I will use high dosages temporarily to get the infection under control. Many times I will use 200,000 to 300,000 IUs for a couple of days, as it helps adults recover from certain viruses quickly. With children, I would never recommend dosages that high. I know that doctors are taught that vitamin A is dangerous and they scare people away from using it. It is not dangerous when the high dosages are only used temporarily. Anything has the potential to be toxic in high enough quantities, including air and water. On a regular basis, 5,000 to 25,000 IUs suffices most of the time. There are herbs high in vitamin A as well. Alfalfa and parsley are two of my favorite herbs because they are so versatile. Alfalfa is wonderful as a kidney support. It is also high in vitamin K which benefits those with arthritis in their joints. It is a great "feel good" tonic. Parsley is also good for the kidneys and urinary tract as well as the lungs.

Dysbiosis

Dysbiosis is such a common problem that I assume everyone has it unless I get an indication otherwise. It is an imbalance in the ecological system in the gut. There should be at least 85% friendly bacteria in the gut versus unfriendly bacteria. Besides bacteria, there can be yeast and fungal overgrowth. There can also be parasites present. Berberine can help eradicate bad bacteria, as can grapefruit seed extract. Garlic, oregano, black walnut, aloe vera, and artemesia anua can all be helpful to eliminate the overgrowth of undesirable elements. Once pathogenic organisms have been eliminated (usually two to three months), high quality probiotics to pump good bacteria back into the intestines are beneficial. It does not hurt to do both at the same time, but typically I will eradicate the bad bacteria first and then balance with friendly bacteria.

There may be obvious discomfort with dysbiosis, but not always. There may also be constipation or diarrhea. Constipation may be relieved with the herbs cascara sagrada, senna, or fennel. Magnesium can also help. I suggest each of these be taken at night before bed. Magnesium will also help you to sleep better as it has a relaxing effect. Pears are a good food for eliminating constipation. Also, it is important to make sure there is enough vegetable fiber in the diet and water intake is sufficient. Drinking a cool glass of water first thing in the morning can stimulate the urge to eliminate. Too much magnesium will cause diarrhea, so the feedback given by the body will help determine the best dosage. If diarrhea is a problem, probiotics will usually help. I have also seen cooling herbs like isatis tinctoria be beneficial, as well as colostrum. The old folk remedy of drinking rice water also works very well. Acacia, grapefruit seed extract, and goldenseal can also help diarrhea.

High blood pressure

High blood pressure (HBP) is a $20 billion a year problem, or profit center, depending on your perspective. Over fifty million people in the U.S. have blood pressure which is considered to be high; however, there is a lot of disagreement about what normal should be. It is widely stated that HBP is a disease, and if you have it, you need to be on medication the rest of your life, yet neither of these statements are true.

As I mentioned previously, HBP is a symptom of a problem in the pumps, pipes, or filters in the body. Symptoms can include headaches, confusion, chest pain, nose bleeds, irregular heartbeat, buzzing in the ears, nausea, and shortness of breath. Whatever is the cause, the result is too much internal pressure. Normalizing weight, avoiding white sugar, flour, and table salt, eliminating caffeine, and decreasing stress can help. Increasing potassium can sometimes be very effective. Excellent to combat high blood pressure are celery juice, beet juice, and blueberries. Other aids include magnesium, hawthorn, coenzyme Q10, vitamin D, L-arginine, and bonito peptides. A sensible exercise program three or four times per week should be included with whatever else is employed.

Cardiovascular disease

Cardiovascular disease is a top killer in the U.S. with congestive heart failure at epidemic levels and rising. Remember, the heart is a muscle, and muscles need certain ingredients to make energy. There is no drug that can help make muscle energy. Coenzyme Q10 is one of the major players. As I previously mentioned, there are certain medications, like cholesterol-lowering statin drugs, that interfere with coenzyme Q10 production in the liver. I do not believe it is a coincidence that as prescriptions have increased for these drugs so has the incidence of congestive heart failure. If you're taking cholesterol lowering medication, particularly statin drugs, at the very least you should be supplementing with coenzyme Q10.

A healthy body requires good fats, so essential fatty acids (EFAs) are needed. That's right, I said it! These fats are essential. To transport EFAs into the part of the cell where energy is made, the mitochondria, L-carnitine is needed. Vitamin B1 (thiamin) has a stimulatory effect on the nervous system and helps convert glucose to energy. D-Ribose is a sugar that also helps with muscle energy. It is a constituent of the citric acid cycle where ATP (energy) is produced in the body. I have seen it be very beneficial to heart patients.

A number of supplements are beneficial for your cardiovascular system. Hawthorn is a marvelous herb for the heart and circulatory system. Remember the movie *Seabiscuit?* A hawthorn poultice wrapped around the horse's leg helped it to heal. If there is clogging of arteries, the enzyme nattokinase has demonstrated the ability to digest the debris and improve circulation. Nattokinase has been used in other parts of the world for circulation problems for some time.

Simple, ordinary beverages are also great. A good drink for the circulatory system is grape juice. Another excellent drink is beet juice. Beet juice has been shown to decrease the oxygen requirement of the body with moderate exercise. The net effect is an increase in endurance.

Potassium and magnesium are two important minerals for cardiovascular health. Both can be depleted under stress and cause serious heart problems if levels are too low. Again, with over three hundred and fifty different metabolic pathways requiring magnesium, it is time to recognize how valuable it really is. It benefits nerve flow to the heart, prevents vasoconstriction, and can help many people heal from heart arrhythmias.

There are a number of great food sources for potassium. Most people think bananas are the best source of potassium. They average about 40 mg each, yet it is not unusual for someone to need as much as 2,000 mg per day. That is a lot of bananas. Then you have to contend with the high sugar content of the bananas, so moderation is best when it comes to this delicious fruit. Green vegetables make a better potassium source. Juicing vegetables, being sure to use a lot of celery, is an excellent way to go. By the way, a high level of potassium on a blood test does not mean someone has too much. I have seen many people who were told not to take any potassium. If they are on potassium-depleting medicines, like some diuretics, and ill-advisably not taking any, it could be a recipe for trouble. High potassium levels can be an indication of high stress and perhaps too much sugar in the diet. Usually the herb licorice will bring down the high potassium levels.

Antiaging support
There are some great tonics that can help maintain a feeling of youth and actually looking younger. Antioxidants are a good place to start to keep inflammation in check. Astaxanthin is

a carotenoid that is one of the strongest antioxidants. In fact, it is 6,000 times stronger than vitamin C as an antioxidant. It is great for keeping the skin and hair looking young. It also increases endurance and muscle recovery time. It helps visual acuity and increases circulation.

Resveratrol is a very good anti-aging remedy. Resveratrol is what gives red wine its good name. The only problem is, to get the true health benefits, you would have to drink so much red wine that the harmful effects would greatly outweigh any benefit. Resveratrol may benefit one's energy, but it is also a very potent antioxidant. Resveratrol triggers the same biochemical reaction as calorie reduction, which has been shown to increase life span.

Keeping hormones balanced is powerful anti-aging therapy. Pregnenolone is the basic ingredient the body uses to make hormones. It has a great balancing effect without the risk of throwing some hormones out of balance by supplementing others. I have seen many thyroid and sex hormone imbalances corrected with pregnenolone supplementation.

DHEA is another hormone support. From DHEA (dehydroepiendosterone) the sex hormones are made. DHEA is made by the adrenal glands, and scientists still have not figured out all that it does. Our production decreases as we get older. Low DHEA levels are associated with many problems, including breast cancer. A common ratio that becomes off balance as we age is that of cortisol and DHEA. Cortisol is a stress hormone and, if secreted too much, it causes all kinds of problems. Increased inflammation, liver and kidney stress, brain issues, like memory loss, ulcerative colitis, and decreased immunity are not uncommon, as well as suppressed DHEA. A low daily dose of DHEA (5 to 10 mg) can help with energy, libido, and increase bone density. It has also been shown that meditation can raise DHEA levels as well.

With women, red clover and black cohosh are two herbs I use commonly. They are particularly effective in balancing estrogen levels. Tulsi is an adaptogen that can balance the entire endocrine system. For males, velvet deer antler, tongkat ali, and tribulus can help with increasing testosterone levels and boosting energy. For benign prostate support saw palmetto, nettles, pygeum, and pumpkin seed can be very beneficial. DHEA and pregnenolone are also beneficial to men as well as women.

Taking a collagen supplement daily is one of the most valuable health tips I can suggest. Here is why I say that. Collagen is the largest and most abundant protein in our body. It makes up 65% of our total protein. Collagen is the connective tissue for almost all of our body structures. As we age, collagen production drops off, and any of our systems may be affected. An example of collagen depletion appears in the drooping of our skin and muscles as we age. Decreased collagen causes instability and weakness of our organs, and has an effect on bones ligaments and tendons. Cartilage becomes thinner and weaker at the joints. Consequently, the joint may become problematic. Collagen affects our bone density as well. Joints and ligaments become weaker and less elastic. Cartilage becomes thinner and weaker at the joints.

Collagen supplementation can help with lean muscle gain and tone, joint rebuilding, hair and nail strength, increased energy, and strengthening and building organs. Problems that can be helped include osteoporosis, high blood pressure, arthritis, bladder weakness, autoimmune conditions, shallow breathing, skin problems, and weak nails. Using collagen gives the body the raw material it needs to repair and rebuild. This means that pain relief comes about because the body is healing, a stark contrast from the pain medications and anti-inflammatories, which are symptomatically oriented and promote destructive processes in the long run. With collagen, the body prioritizes where it is needed. We are simply giving it the resources it needs to heal. Collagen is one of the best joint healing, as well as anti-aging substances we can take.

Keeping glutathione levels up is essential to a long healthy life. It is one of the best bio markers of good health. The eighty-year-old with the highest glutathione level will be the healthiest one. For glutathione to be made there are certain ingredients necessary. Two enzymatic pathways are precursors to glutathione synthesis. One is selenium dependent and the other is riboflavin (vitamin B2) dependent. There are other precursors as well, including N-acetyl-cysteine (NAC), lipoic acid, whey protein, and turmeric. It can be very healing at the cellular level.

To keep energy and vitality up, stress must not win the battle. We need to feed our bodies with nutrient dense foods. Some foods are actually classified as "superfoods" for their ability to give us great energy. I always tell patients that are busy and trying to accomplish a lot in their life to treat themselves like a valued race car. How would you do that? You keep it finely tuned, get any problems taken care of right away, and put in the best fuel possible.

Treat yourself the same way. Super green foods are excellent. Wheat grass, spirulina, and chlorella are some of my favorites. Besides providing energy, they have detoxifying capabilities, and chlorella can also help with arthritis pain. Chlorella is very high in chlorophyll which makes it good for the intestines as well.

Some of the other benefits of chlorella are:

- Boosts immunity
- Increases energy
- Good source of amino acids
- Heavy metal detoxification
- Improves blood pressure
- Excellent source of antioxidants
- Lowers triglyceride levels
- Improved insulin sensitivity
- Aids digestion

Other superfoods are chia seeds and maca. The Tarahamara Indians of Northern Mexico are the best long distance runners in the world. Chia seeds are one of their staples. It is not uncommon for them to do 100 mile runs. They communicate amongst the villages of Copper Canyon by running. They are not eating American fast food that would sap their energy. Their tortillas are made from non-GMO corn, fresh and loaded with nutrition.

Maca is another excellent superfood. The Mayans and Aztecs reportedly ate maca which explains in part the tremendous endurance and stamina these people had. I like organic Peruvian maca. You can feel the energizing effect almost immediately after taking it.

Whatever the condition, I believe nature has a remedy for it. I said that once at a talk I was giving, and someone in the audience responded, *"Doesn't something like a severe fracture require medical intervention or perhaps surgery?"* I replied, *"That is true, however, there are still natural remedies that can be utilized that will expedite the healing a great deal."* In the case of fractures, there are herbs like boneset and cissus quadrangularis that help bone to heal. The herb Solomen's Seal helps the tendons and ligaments heal. Calcium hydroxyapatite along with vitamin K2, boron, manganese, and magnesium can also be supportive for bone healing. If surgery becomes necessary, proteolytic enzymes can help speed up the repair and recovery process, and in some cases can increase healing by at least half the time.

For every ailment, natural remedies can be utilized for faster healing, to decrease the amount of pharmaceuticals needed, or resolve the condition. There will always be a place for drugs and surgery, but for health and healing think *natural*.

chapter SIX

BEYOND FOOD

What we eat is extremely important to our health, but it is only part of the story. How the body handles the food determines how much benefit we receive from it. I will elaborate on that more, but first, I want to talk about diet. By diet, I am referring to what we choose to eat, instead of restricting calories for weight loss or another goal. As a rule, I try to keep things simple and easy to understand.

There is much conflicting information out there, with the result a confused public. The books that promote "the best diet" or "the only way we should eat" I usually do not recommend. The approach that for a certain blood type there is a specific dietary protocol to follow does not always work clinically either. There are many other factors to consider. The diet being promoted may have helped the author get healthy, but one size does not fit all. I will assure you that just as many people will have negative results as are helped by any given program.

Here are six basic rules regarding food. Then I will discuss the biggest factor people miss. It is at least as important as the diet itself.

1. Eat real food. It is simple yet today most people do not know what real food is. The Standard American Diet (SAD) is high in processed foods, sugar, white flour, and chemical additives, and low in nutrition and practically devoid of healthy fruits and vegetables. This diet is a failure and will eventually lead to health problems.

The top selling items in grocery stores are not foods. I have seen people in the grocery store with carts overflowing and not have a real food item in them. Some items found in a grocery store that are not real food include sodas, deli meats, processed milk, pastries, fake butter, artificial sugars, enriched flour products like most pastas, and breads, and most boxed breakfast cereals.

There is a good reason to eat real food. Very simply, the body requires it to function. Deprived of this requirement, it is only a matter of time before health issues manifest.

When people eat deficient or processed foods, these foods actually rob the body of the very nutrients that are removed during processing, nutrients that exist within these foods in their natural state.

For example, whole sugar cane is high in several B vitamins and minerals like chromium and magnesium, which are all necessary for the body to utilize sugar. When processed into refined white sugar, all these nutrients are taken out. In order for the body to digest refined sugar, these very same nutrients and enzymes are then withdrawn from the body when the processed product is ingested. *This is how a processed diet causes nutritional deficiencies and is one of the biggest missed laws of nutrition there is.*

The best foods are live foods. A live food will spoil in time. That is what should happen. If a food can sit on a grocery shelf for six months, it is not live. You get the idea. Real foods include fruits and vegetables (organic when possible), whole grains, natural meats, and wild fish. Yet when I look at what many people eat every day, processed foods and refined carbohydrates prevail. Around the country, most cities look alike anymore with a fast food restaurant on nearly every corner.

In addition to being poor quality food, fast food is full of harmful chemicals like MSG, and artificial colors and flavors. It astounds me that with all the laws and regulations that exist in this country, it is still allowable to put MSG in food.

The recent revelation, first uncovered and reported in the *Natural News* newsletter, that ammonia is mixed in with fast food hamburgers to sterilize the meat, and another recent discovery that there is a meat "glue" designed to make cuts of meat look higher quality, makes me wonder what else is in food we do not know about yet. This is done with the government's approval. Their idea of food safety is to kill the food, sterilize, pasteurize, and irradiate it. Then it is safe to eat.

What would we ever do without the government to protect us? Searching the Internet for the "world's first bionic burger" will make you wonder what consuming a burger that will not spoil after eighteen years (and counting) will do to your body. The only redeeming factor I can think of is after people die they will already be preserved and ready for burial. I read that the main vitamin C source for teenagers is french fries, which are mainly purchased at fast food restaurants. I can't believe there is any vitamin C left after all that cooking in heated oil, but even if there were, what a trade off: a little vitamin C for increasing your cancer risk dramatically.

The main reason to eat real food is that it is already balanced perfectly in its natural state. Nature cannot be improved on. The notion that eggs raise cholesterol levels for example, preys on the nutritional ignorance of the public. While eggs do contain cholesterol, they also contain cholesterol mobilizers, like lecithin. That myth was perpetuated to get people to buy artificial egg substitutes that had no positive health benefits whatsoever.

Another example of nature's wisdom is avocados. I hear people state all the time that they won't eat them because of the fat content. Yes, they do contain fats but here is an important point. You *do not* get fat on natural fats. Also, avocados are high in the enzyme lipase, which helps to digest fat. Natural fats are important to good health. Natural fats are extremely important to make hormones in the body, for the nervous system, and the brain requires them for optimal functioning. Other great sources of natural fats are walnuts, flax, and chia seeds.

2. Eat a protein with each meal. If you are physically active you need to increase your protein intake. The body needs protein to repair, carry nutrients to their destinations, and detoxify. It has been shown that protein deprivation for only twenty four hours can stress the liver. Good protein sources include natural meats, chicken, eggs, cottage cheese, nuts and seeds, whey, and vegan protein supplements from, rice, hemp, or pea. Always buy organic when it is available. I am not including soy here, although it is widely available. Most soy is genetically altered (GMO) and is also one of the most insecticide-sprayed crops in the country, along with cotton and corn.

3. Complex carbohydrates only. Everyone benefits by removing refined carbohydrates from the diet. Rarely should cakes, pastries, and other refined wheat products be consumed. I limit them to birthday parties only. Refined sugar has no nutrition and no health benefits. High intake is correlated to many health problems, from diabetes, to heart disease, to cancer.

My favorite complex carbohydrates are whole grain rice, sweet potatoes, and yams. All are nutrient and fiber rich and the latter two are good for the hormonal system. If pasta is desired, I get the non-wheat pastas or those made in Italy. Italian pastas are often made from higher quality wheat and are minimally processed. In many products made from commercial wheat flour, most of the nutrients are removed during the refining process. Also much wheat has been in storage for at least two years before it is turned into a wheat product and sold commercially. So, look for breads that are made with organic wheat berries, rather than wheat flour.

Everybody is also better off removing soft drinks from their diet. There is no redeeming feature to these sodas. Sales continue to increase each year. They are the preferred drink of many but especially so among our youth. They are one of the biggest sources of sugar and high fructose corn syrup, which tops the list of health destroyers.

I do not recommend a diet high in high fructose corn syrup because it disrupts appetite control, is made from genetically modified corn, and has been shown to be high in mercury. There are healthier, natural sweeteners available. The really bad news is that high fructose corn syrup is the number one calorie source for kids.

I also do not recommend diet drinks as a good option. Artificial sugars are very harmful substances to put in the body. They are toxic to the liver and brain and do not help you lose weight. The suggestion that they help weight loss is a cruel joke being played on our population.

4. Time of day matters. It is best to eat a hearty breakfast and lunch and go lighter in the evening. Your digestive system is at its best between 10:00 a.m. and 2:00 p.m. That would be the ideal time frame to eat most of the day's food intake. Eating much later puts stress on the body's digestive system and has negative consequences. Eating right before bed is especially not good, particularly if primarily carbohydrates are being consumed. This puts us on a fast track for weight gain, hormone imbalance (particularly leptin), and blood sugar imbalances.

5. When increasing protein intake, be sure to increase water. The idea that protein can be stressful to the kidneys is only partly true. Actually, anything the body can't digest can affect the kidneys, but dehydration is usually the culprit. Also, consuming meals with a meat protein should be combined with vegetables. The rule is: The more meat being consumed, whatever the source, the more vegetables should be included.

6. Water, water, water! Did I mention the importance of drinking adequate water? Water should be the beverage of choice. Most people are dehydrated and water is the only solution. My recommendation is to drink one half of your body weight in ounces of water per day. Also, go easy on the diuretics like caffeine and sugar. Water is needed to flush toxins from the body, helps all systems function, like the brain, and helps normalize blood sugar. Many people think that any liquid counts toward hydration. However, in reality, any drink made of water, the body construes as food. Some drinks, like coffee, tea or sodas, actually dehydrate the body. For example, every cup of coffee depletes the body of two cups of water metabolically.

That is about it. There is nothing complicated or new about these recommendations. They are simple, yet very few of us follow them. When we do, body weight normalizes, energy levels rise, moods change for the better, and blood test results improve.

If people are used to a hugely processed diet, they may have to make changes in a series of steps. For example, I had a patient who literally drank fifty cups of coffee a day. I did not tell him to stop all coffee right away. That would have been too stressful, and he probably would have stopped trying and resumed his old habits. I had him gradually decrease the coffee consumption and increase his water intake. We also looked at how he may have been dealing with stress in inappropriate ways by using coffee as a crutch. It was difficult, but he was successful. He gradually reduced his intake, and needed to support his adrenals, which were completely depleted. We also looked at what triggered his stress and found better ways to encourage him to handle this. I was able to show him that the excess coffee intake was also contributing to a pain in his mid back.

Food choices are important, but even if the diet is perfect, the body must be able to digest and metabolize the food. Otherwise, there is limited nutritional benefit from the food consumed. This is the biggest factor that diet programs miss:

It doesn't matter how correct the diet is. If the body cannot digest what is consumed, there is little or no nutritional benefit from eating.

Very importantly, when there are digestive issues or incompetencies, musculoskeletal complaints will manifest. The nerves that innervate the digestive area that is stressed will become irritated and cause the muscles sharing the same nerve supply to contract, which results in pain. The musculoskeletal complaints can be in the spine (at the spinal source of the involved nerve) or at the muscle attachment sites. A classic sign of chronic digestive issues is called a Pottinger's Saucer, in which the spine between the shoulder blades scoops in. Stomach, gall bladder, and pancreatic stress can manifest as spinal discomfort in the mid-thoracic region, between or slightly below the shoulder blades

Digestive difficulties are so common I assume every adult and most children who come into my office have them, whether they have obvious complaints or not.

Here is a brief summary of the digestive process, so you can see why it is so important:

- Digestion begins in the mouth with chewing. There are enzymes secreted by the salivary glands, which include amylase, lipase, and some protease. These enzymes, combined with the enzymes that may be present in the food, start the predigestion process.
- This process continues in the upper part of the stomach while the acidifying begins in the stomach with the secreting of hydrochloric acid via the parietal cells of the stomach.
- When the pH of the stomach drops to three or below, in normal digestion, the enzyme pepsin is released from pepsinogen and its main job is protein digestion. This acid pH temporarily deactivates the other enzymes.
- The stomach contents move into the upper part of the small intestine (the duodenum) and the enzymes are re-activated in an alkaline environment. Here, pancreatic enzymes join the party as does bile from the gall bladder.
- The next part of the small intestine (the jeju-

num) is where sugars are digested by disaccharidases if the intestines are healthy and functioning well. The small intestines are where most nutrients are absorbed.

The gall bladder is another very important digestive player:

- The gall bladder is a small organ next to the liver, whose job is to hold bile after the liver produces it. Bile is secreted into the upper part of the small intestines during digestion.
- Bile acts as a detergent, which emulsifies fats and facilitates the absorption of cholesterol.
- If there are not enough bile salts, much of the important, nourishing fats are lost in the elimination process via bowel movements. If this goes on long enough, deficiencies occur in fat-soluble nutrients like vitamins A, D, E, and K.

Many people have gall bladder stress that causes either indigestion or pain. Gall stones are one of the main reasons for removing the gall bladder. Gall stones form if there are not enough bile salts and the cholesterol separates, or due to chronic dehydration or acidity. Gall stones do not have to be present to have gall bladder stress, however. Certain food sensitivities can trigger gall bladder discomfort. Some common foods that trigger this are milk, wheat, and chocolate. If symptoms have started, fried foods, all oils, raw onions, processed cane sugar, and high fat foods should be avoided.

Sadly, hundreds of thousands of gall bladders are removed each year. Make no mistake, gall bladder dysfunction can make one feel quite sick, but most can remedy the problem without removing it and will benefit tremendously from attempting natural remedies to alleviate their discomfort before considering drastic surgical options.

Other circumstances that lead to digestive problems are illness and medicines. Recurrent antibiotic use can cause problems. The depletion of the body's friendly bacteria sets one up for opportunistic pathogens to get a foothold. Antibiotics also stress the spleen, which plays a role in digestion, immunity, and energy production. I find it troubling that with all the talk of problems from antibiotic overuse (even in the mainstream media); I do not see a lot of change clinically. As I stated previously, people are still being prescribed antibiotics for non-bacterial infections. Remember, antibiotics are only effective against bacteria and they are not nearly as effective as they used to be.

Many of our digestive problems begin in childhood when we are fed the wrong foods too early in life. Many mothers start their children on grains too soon. The easiest foods to digest should be given first: pureed fruits, then vegetables, and only when there are teeth present. Grains should be the last foods introduced, not the first, and wheat flour products are best avoided. Rice would be a better choice.

There are many other causes of digestive inefficiencies, but for children probably the biggest is not being breast fed. I assume that most people who were not breastfed have an intestinal weakness. Mother's milk has so many wonderful nutrients in it and should always be given when possible. Colostrum in the first milk is very important for intestinal and immune health. To compound the problem, formula is usually substituted and mixed with processed cow's milk. To say this is less than sufficient to nourish an infant is an understatement.

When I was a child, mothers were told formula was actually superior to their own milk. Unbelievable, yet most women went along with it because it was their doctor's advice. In the years that followed, there was a world conference to promote breast feeding as the best way to feed an infant. Every country signed the resolution except the U.S. Again, our government seemed to be more concerned about corporate interests than the health of U.S. children.

Many of the top selling infant formulas contain up to 52% sugar and processed ingredients. I do not believe this gives children a healthy beginning. Processed cow's milk is not a healthy food for children either. It is very hard to digest and sets children up for health issues down the road. Even a calf will not thrive on drinking processed cow's milk.

As I write this, the government has waged war on the sale of raw (unpasteurized) milk. They make it clear they do not want it sold, even though it is healthier than processed milk. The primary argument is that it can become contaminated more easily. Can it become contaminated? Sure. So can processed milk. If left out of the refrigerator, the pasteurized milk will rot and become unfit to drink. Contaminated pasteurized milk can actually be more dangerous because there are no enzymes present to neutralize the pathogens. Raw milk will sour and actually remains a healthy food.

For adults, continually eating the wrong foods, a high sugar and wheat intake, and drinking too much alcohol or caffeine, will contribute to digestion problems. The body will go into an adaptive mode and rob from one system to feed another in an effort to sustain life. This innate survival mechanism is built into the miraculous human body. Organs and systems that are essential for life, like the brain, nervous system, and liver, will take precedence over less important systems and functions. For example, the reproductive system after age 35 is not considered essential and can be one of the first systems sacrificed. The problem is, after a while, the body may run out of systems to borrow from because its tank is on empty, which puts people on a fast track to declining health.

The importance of enzymes:

The bottom line is this, and it bears repeating: *It does not matter how good the diet is if the body cannot digest and metabolize the food.* Whatever the body can't digest will create stress and nutritional deficiencies. The solution to this problem is to take enzymes. Enzymes are special proteins that make life happen by their ability to digest food and produce energy. To have healthy organ and intestinal systems, the body requires enzymes for digestion. The importance of enzymes cannot be overstated. Without them, functioning suffers and can stop altogether. Since most people are both depleting their enzymes and not consuming enough, this pattern cannot continue indefinitely without health problems manifesting. Vitamins and minerals are very important, but again, if enzymes are not present to drive the biochemical reactions, they will not be successful in aiding health.

There are many different enzymes, but the main types include food, pancreatic, and metabolic enzymes. The body makes over a thousand metabolic enzymes to run the inner workings. Virtually every bodily function requires these enzymes. As I mentioned previously, during digestion pancreatic enzymes are secreted by the pancreas into the upper part of the small intestine to continue the digestive process that actually began in the mouth with chewing. Food and plant enzymes work in a broader pH range than pancreatic enzymes. Outside of their required pH range for functioning, they are deactivated (not destroyed). They can reactivate in their needed pH environment. Food enzymes are present in live food, like fruits and vegetables. Heat destroys enzymes, so the challenge for health-minded people is to make sure we get plenty of non-cooked or non-pasteurized foods daily.

The consequences from not getting plenty of food enzymes in the diet can be severe. The body requires live food sources in order to thrive. To feed a live body only dead food does not serve the body well. Besides not being the best source of nutrition, it actually can stress and deplete the body.

The body, particularly the pancreas, was not meant to supply all of the enzyme requirements it needs. If there is none in the food, predigestion will suffer, meaning the pancreas will need to come to the aid of the digestive process even more by supplying more enzymes. If this occurs every day, week, and year, the pancreas will become stressed and may actually have to borrow from other enzyme systems to do its job. This could lead to metabolic stress as well. When there is stress to an organ, it will swell. Upon autopsy, almost every American has a hypertrophied (swollen) pancreas. What does that say about the typical American diet and the ability to digest this food?

The good news is that food enzyme supplements are available. Taken before meals they help predigest food, make the digestive process easier, help the body get more nutrition from food, and spare the pancreas. If you forget to take them before, there is still a benefit to taking them up to 20 minutes after a meal. The benefit decreases with the length of time after the meal.

I do not believe that is a substitute for eating plenty of live foods, but using food enzymes is certainly a way to boost overall health. Not doing so is to gamble with your health. All you have to do is look at the health statistics in the U.S. and you quickly realize we have a major crisis happening. The U.S. has the worst health statistics of any industrialized country, and we keep promoting all the things that got us into that situation. Live food will not be an option if we stay on this absolutely insane course.

A case can be made that many health issues are related to an enzyme deficiency. For example, a protease deficiency can cause:

- Someone who is deficient in protease, which digests proteins, may have a compromised immune system and chronic infections may result. Swelling of the feet or hands, called edema, may also be present.
- Colon toxicity from undigested proteins can cause constipation, contribute to appendicitis, and even promote cancer.
- Hypoglycemia (low blood sugar) can be caused by a protease deficiency, since half the protein digested is converted to sugar.
- Protein carries calcium in the blood, so many of the calcium metabolism problems like osteoporosis, disc problems, and osteoarthritis can actually be protease deficiency symptoms.
- Any conditions that ice would benefit, specifically heat symptoms, are generally helped with protease. It helps with post-surgical recovery to boost the immune system.
- Bacterial infections can also be particularly helped with protease. Protease supplements should be taken with meals to aid protein digestion. They may also be taken between meals to combat inflammatory issues, particularly soft tissue injuries.

The enzyme amylase digests carbohydrates, so they are broken down into smaller molecules that the body can use. Many people who overdo carbohydrates are actually fat intolerant. This is how one digestive difficulty can create another. There is a reason why people will have a particular affinity for a type of food. The body needs certain nutrients, so it creates a craving for them. However when the body can't digest the food, the craving is not satisfied, and people will still crave what they can't digest.

Lipase is the enzyme that digests fats. People who have a lipase deficiency may have high triglycerides, high blood pressure, difficulty losing weight, or be deficient in fat-soluble nutrients. Diabetics, as a rule, have a problem digesting fats which, in turn, interferes with the movement of glucose inside the cell by insulin. Taking supplements with meals can aid fat digestion. People without gall bladders would also benefit from an ox bile supplement to emulsify fats first, so lipase can then digest them.

Pancreatic enzymes work in the small intestine and can be taken after or in between meals. If taken in between meals they can tonify the digestive system and also be beneficial as an anti-inflammatory.

Often I get the question of how do we run into enzyme deficiencies? The quality of the diet must be examined first. Eating enzyme deficient foods depletes the body. A food is enzyme deficient if it can sit on a shelf for months without spoiling, whether in a box, jar, or can, or if it has been exposed to high temperatures. Enzymes are the enemy of food processing. They must be destroyed to preserve the food from spoiling.

The depletion of these enzymes is most affected by the over-consumption of refined sugars. The per capita sugar consumption in the U.S. is the highest in the world, over

150 pounds per year. The body simply can't handle that much. Disaccharidases, the enzymes which digest sugars, do their digesting in the small intestine. This is also where 95% of the body's serotonin is made. Serotonin imbalances can create mood swings, bipolar problems, and obsessive-compulsive disorders.

The health consequences, both mentally and physically from this dietary error of sugar overconsumption are enormous. Everything from heart disease to depression is a possibility. Diseases like cancer are fed by sugar. The thyroid gland can turn sluggish because of too much sugar. Attention Deficit Disorder, panic attacks, and aggressive behaviors are also on the rise. It is no coincidence that these problems have become more prevalent in correlation with increased sugar intake.

An enzyme deficiency, which can result in undigested foods, can also promote yeast and fungal overgrowth. This problem is particularly aggravated by the inability to digest sugars. Sugar feeds pathogenic organisms and creates a very unhealthy environment at the cellular level, partly due to its acidity. Yeast is a toxin that makes other toxic byproducts which wreak havoc on the body, stressing the liver, affecting the brain, and inflaming the sinuses.

Besides the food itself, we are continually bombarded with other circumstances that deplete enzymes. Here are a few more:

1. Cooking at high temperatures. Temperatures over 118° F will kill enzymes. Heat processing like pasteurization will destroy enzymes. In fact, when milk is pasteurized, the process is not considered complete until the enzyme phosphatase is no longer present.

2. Pesticides and other chemicals. Pesticides work by destroying enzymes that control the nervous system as well as cellular functioning. Even very small amounts can be hazardous. With over a billion pounds (and growing) being sprayed each year in the U.S., this is a huge problem. Toxic chemicals in the home should be avoided. Insecticides and toxic cleaning chemicals should not be used. You do not have to eat something for it to affect your body. Contact with your skin or inhaling fumes can be enough to do damage. For these reasons, it is also a good idea to avoid fluoridated and chlorinated water.

3. Food irradiation destroys enzymes as well as other nutrients. It does kill some harmful bacteria, but not all. The concept of using radioactive waste material to keep our food safe seems irrational to me.

4. Microwave ovens. These are a fast, efficient way to destroy your food. When you microwave food, you kill it, plain and simple. For example, if you planted a sprouting potato in the ground it would grow. Take that same potato and microwave it for one minute on high, take it out, plant it and nothing will ever happen. Think about putting that same dead food in your body. What good could possibly result from that?

The importance of enzymes and proper digestion cannot be stressed enough. I have witnessed rapid relief of stomach pain, diarrhea, constipation, Crohn's disease, and ulcerative colitis, by changing the diet and aiding the functioning of the digestive process.

In the absence of such acute symptoms, when efficient digestion is promoted, people over time simply feel better in a myriad of ways. They become healthier, as the body receives more nutrition from the food consumed. It is one of the most important elements to healthier aging and turning back the clock.

People feel better and are actually functioning with more youthfulness at greater physical ages. I can honestly say that when it comes to nutrition, utilizing enzymes along with proper food sources is as close to "the miracle cure" as it gets.

chapter SEVEN

THE TURN BACK THE CLOCK MINDSET

To become youthful requires the right mindset. Having this mindset will keep you inspired to take the necessary steps to make it all happen and, at the same time, add to your fulfillment in life.

To begin with, be realistic about where you are right now. Is your weight where you want it? How is your energy? Do you feel excited about life, or has life beaten you down? What do your blood test results reveal? Do you have goals that you are striving to achieve? Are you taking prescription drugs for any medical condition?

I recommend you focus on improvement in any area that is not satisfactory to you – then choose one at a time. Once you decide what you want to improve, write it down and commit to accomplishing the goal. This is very simple, yet very few people will get this far. However, *you* can, and will, if you just commit to doing it. That is the first and most important step.

It is very common for self-sabotage to begin immediately. Be careful not to undermine yourself before you begin. Be aware that this can happen, and you might need to refocus. In some cases, you might need to refocus often, or even continually. This does not mean to judge yourself as being less than just fine as you are. Who you are at the deepest level is already perfect. Your waistline is not who you are.

This new mindset is about staying healthy and vital so your physical and emotional experience is as good as possible while you are here. As the late Jim Rohn used to say, *"Life is about experiences and the intensity of those experiences."* Obviously you can have more and better experiences when you are feeling good. Often people will talk about how they want to feel better, have more energy, and do more of something. Yet talking is as far as most will go.

There are essentially two types of people: talkers and doers. Guess what there are more of? If you guessed talkers, you are right by far.

Commit to being a doer.

Once you take the first step by actually acting on a goal, you have entered the realm of "the doers club." It is an exclusive group of only a very small percentage of the population, not more than 3%. Once you begin, you will wonder why everyone is not doing what you are, and why you did not begin sooner. My suggestion is that you do not spend much time wondering. What you are doing now is important, not what you did in the past. Do not waste time figuring out why people do (or don't do) what they talk about.

"Some will and some won't. Trying to figure out why is a waste of time." — Jim Rohn

It is important to understand some of the roadblocks. At some point if you are feeling stalled, you may recognize one of these issues is surfacing. I have observed many people over the years that would come into my office, ask and pay for advice, then leave and not do anything. I never could understand why. So many times it was not difficult to implement the changes I recommended, and I knew they would benefit tremendously. However, they chose to do nothing, and of course, nothing changed in their lives.

That used to frustrate me until I understood why it is not easy for people to make changes. Perhaps you will recognize some of these traits in yourself. I know I did. That is a good thing. With that awareness and understanding you can now take specific steps to change your life. You can become part of that "doer" group, an exclusive club to which you will be proud to belong.

Here are six reasons people do not take action, but *you* can.

1. Get serious and get started. The first roadblock to making improvements is that many people simply are not serious about it. They might talk about it, wish, and hope, but deep down the desire is not there. For many their favorite word is "someday." Someday I am going to start exercising. Someday I will eat healthier. Someday. Someday rarely comes. Do not let someday be your mantra. Be honest with yourself. Do you really want to feel and look better and increase your odds of a longer and healthier life? If so, create a strong desire to do what is necessary to achieve your goals. Commit to not giving up. My friend and mentor Keith Leon teaches, *"The only way to finish is to get started."* I agree.

2. Have a reason to change. Many people do not have strong reasons to change. Yes, they know they should do something, but without strong enough reasons to commit to a goal, most won't stay with it. Sometimes desperation sets in after a health crisis, for example. Facing their mortality, I have seen people effect remarkable turn-arounds very quickly because they had reasons to live. In my experience, the best reasons reach beyond your personal desires. To get healthier to watch grandchildren grow up is more potent than the goal of just getting a blood pressure reading down. I asked a gentleman with crippling arthritis what he would like to accomplish. He replied, *"I would love to dance with my wife again."* That is a powerful reason to strive for improvement. That is what you need.

3. Educate yourself. Regarding health, many people are confused by all the conflicting information out there. Their reaction is to do nothing because they are uncertain what advice to follow. This is understandable; however, there are a few very important, simple rules, many of which I have outlined in this book. My suggestion is start with these basics: Eat real food, take enzymes, increase water intake and vegetables, cut out white sugar, flour and salt, start exercising, and monitor your thoughts.

Make sure you get information from credible sources. Television is not generally one of them. I remember a few years ago the head of a large federal bureaucracy was on *The Larry King Show*. Larry King asked him what people should believe, considering there was so much contradictory information out there. This politician, without missing a beat, responded that his agency would *tell* the public what was good for them, and they could simply trust him and his agency. If that does not send shivers down your spine, it should. I did my research and knew this same federal agency had allowed MSG into food, food dyes that are known carcinogens, and sterilizing fast food hamburgers with ammonia. Who would consider them a credible source of good health information?

Once you have a basic understanding of health and nutrition, you can quickly see through some of the malicious propaganda that consistently bombards us via the media. The next time you see someone with a Ph.D. telling you that irradiating food does nothing to the food you will know to doubt his credibility. You will know that irradiating food kills the enzymes so it won't spoil, thus giving longer shelf life. In other words, it makes the food dead.

4. Accept responsibility for yourself. Many people, probably even the majority, do not accept responsibility for themselves. They are always looking for somebody, or another entity like a government agency, to either take responsibility or do it for them. Your health is your responsibility and not something you can delegate to others. You can't have somebody else exercise for you. Most do not like the sound of that.

Until you take responsibility for everything in your life, it is unlikely you will take even the first step toward making changes. The person who will not quit smoking or drinking sodas will say things like, *"You've got to die from something."* Isn't that a great philosophy? I remember several years ago I had a patient suffering from severe stomach ulcers. He drank a six pack of Classic Coke a day, a habit he refused to stop. It was easier for him to die than change. I realize that change sometimes requires delving into very deep traumas that are difficult to look at. It is, however, a necessary step toward positive growth.

Not taking responsibility is an easy cop-out. I have noticed this negative attitude is not exclusive to one aspect of a person's life, but tends to prevail over all areas. T. Harv Eker says, *"How you do one thing is how you do everything."* Blaming parents, the government, bad genes, bad luck, or any other external target will not do one thing to further you along life's path or create lasting positive change in life.

5. Expand your beliefs. So many people have limiting beliefs that hold them back. These beliefs become part of the brain and nervous system, and finally become part of the DNA. Here is the kicker. These limiting beliefs, almost always, are not even theirs. They belonged to somebody else, but were accepted without examination. Often these limiting beliefs came from parents, teachers or other authoritative people like politicians, or doctors. People will often base their whole identity or potential, on someone else's belief or opinion.

As Les Brown says so eloquently, *"You never want to base your opinion about yourself on someone else's opinion of you."* I certainly have been guilty of this myself. I was not a good student in high school and I got through college with a lot of studying, but I did not think I could pass certain science or math classes. That was my previous experience, and my belief was supported by teachers and others.

Well, to get into chiropractic college, I was required to take science classes, which included chemistry and physics, when I felt I could barely pass remedial math. I did not have the confidence I could do it based on my previous programming. Yet when I made a commitment to graduate, doors started to open for me, and I received help from people I did not even know. With my strong desire to succeed, and help from these unexpected life experiences, I got through it. The insecurity that I harbored made the whole experience much more stressful than it needed to be, but with my new belief system I came very close to getting a 4.0 grade point average my first quarter and wound up graduating Cum Laude.

Whenever limiting beliefs is the topic, the story of the four-minute mile always comes to mind. For years it was believed that running a mile in under four minutes was impossible. Once it was achieved, however, it was soon common for someone to run a sub-four-minute mile. People will act in accordance to their beliefs. Do not limit your thinking or action because you have limiting beliefs. Dr. Robert Schuller uses the term "possibility thinking." Why be so quick to believe what can't be done? What about all those so-called experts who said a human could not run a sub-four-minute mile?

Today we still have experts endorsing limitations that are just as erroneous. I like how Wayne Dyer responds. He says if you ask an expert for a solution, they will give you one or two absolutes for an answer. Ask a beginner and they will give you all kinds of possibilities. It is best to always ask a beginner, and always be a beginner. You have no idea what you are capable of. Most assuredly, it is much more than you have ever imagined.

We usually let into our lives only what our beliefs allow, regardless of how limiting they are. My personal experience is no exception. I was in the mountains a couple of years ago, fishing the Walker River in a beautiful, large meadow. The sun was coming up over the peaks and it was a brilliant morning. My friend and I were alone. I cast my line for the first time and my fishing lure got stuck in a log. When I yanked the line to pull it out, it shot back at me like a bullet, and the barbed hook lodged deeply into my arm.

I was horrified and convinced this would ruin my trip. After I drove the 27 miles back to town, I got a rude awakening. The hospital had been closed down two years earlier. There were, however, two young paramedics in a trailer at the rear of the hospital. When I showed them my arm, one looked at it and said he could remove the hook. *"The only problem is I don't have any anesthesia,"* he said. Not what I wanted to hear, but I needed his help, so I agreed.

I sat in the little trailer and he started working on the lure in my arm with dental floss. I'm not sure exactly what he was doing because I couldn't bring myself to watch, but I was sure I would wind up with a hole in my arm the size of Texas. After about 20 minutes, the man said, *"On the count of three, I'll give it a tug."* He tugged but the hook did not budge. He asked my permission to try again and then set to work with the dental floss for another 15 minutes. I was surprised that all his work did not hurt as much as I expected, but I still couldn't look. *"On the count of three, I'll give it another tug."* He yanked on the count of two, and the hook popped out easily. I was astonished to see that the only evidence was two tiny red marks on my arm. It wasn't even bleeding. It looked like a magic trick. He even refused to accept payment.

According to my limiting belief, it would have been impossible to remove a barbed fish hook from my arm without being extremely painful, leaving a huge bleeding wound, and costing a lot of money. When I saw the results, I had an immediate expansion of what I believed to be possible. It was a great life lesson. I was grateful for the experience – and for the country doctor's simple but amazingly effective methods.

6. Expect and welcome failure. The fear of failure is one of the biggest obstacles to achievement there is, as we discussed in Chapter 3. It creates a subconscious feeling that it is safer to do nothing. This "I can't" attitude often stems from attempting things as a child and receiving criticism or punishment. After a while the child becomes afraid to attempt new things for fear of the repercussions.

This fear of attempting new things is not limited to children. As adults we are often afraid we will either disappoint others or won't live up to their expectations. Usually we feel something is wrong or defective about us. When we start something new, which then fails, it validates that feeling. We believe that by *not* doing anything we can keep our secret flaws to ourselves (even though they are all in our heads). When we are paralyzed by fears, we guarantee we will not achieve the things we want because we never take action, which validates our beliefs about ourselves. In other words, our erroneous beliefs set up a chain of events that proves us right, even though there is nothing right about it. It is all based on a lie we chose to accept as truth.

The average person will attempt something new *less than one time* in anticipation of failure. The thought of trying new things often paralyzes people. What needs to happen is a total re-framing of what failure means. Failure is something to be welcomed on the pathway to success, rather than something to be feared.

Failure is not a final defeat, but rather a barometer of what is not working. It helps us to get back on track and guides us toward expansion and growth. I like the airplane analogy. How often is an airplane perfectly on course? Most people do not know this, but the answer is hardly ever. The pilot is constantly making adjustments to keep the plane as closely on course as possible. We should be doing the same thing: constantly adjusting, learning, and yes, failing.

It is very important to reframe our perception of fear and failure so it encourages us to take action instead of bringing us down. I admit freely, it took most of my adult life to grasp this concept: It is impossible to succeed without failure. Remember, you can only fail by *not* doing something. It is far better to make an attempt than to not do anything at all. Do not worry about the critics. What I have observed over the years is that most critics do not do anything. They rationalize their inaction by pointing out other people's faults and failures. Do not give the critics one second of your time. They are not worth it. If they ever bring something constructive to the table, then they might earn the right of your attention. However, I would not anticipate that happening.

Successful people fail more because they take more risks. Those who have achieved fantastic levels of success have often failed more than most. Their success has over shadowed their failures so greatly that nobody cares about the failures. Michael Jordan missed twenty nine game winning shots in his career. Does anybody remember? Does anybody care? No. He had so many wins, and had such an exemplary career, that the losses are relegated to the insignificant statistics department. Babe Ruth set a strikeout record the same year he set the home run record. Most people do not know about the strikeouts, and even if they did, they do not care. The trick is to fail forward and keep putting one foot in front of the other, just as Michael Jordan and Babe Ruth did.

Vitality is a reality. If you implement the suggestions presented in the following list, I have no doubt they can propel you to new levels of living and being you'll enjoy. You can actually feel younger and your whole life can change for the better.

Let's explore six topics that will help you become better in every way.

1. Have the right attitude. Simply put, your attitude will determine whether you succeed or fail. Your attitude is a choice. You choose to either have the attitude necessary to accomplish your goals or not. It really is that simple. Decide to have the right attitude. It is not necessary to have a perfect attitude all the time. That is not realistic. To accomplish anything worthwhile you must be motivated to do so. Motivation depends on having the right attitude. Critics (remember those are usually the people not doing anything) are always quick to point out that motivation does not last, and is, therefore, a waste of time. There is some truth to this, but it is often an unfounded excuse to be cynical.

A one-time shot of motivation probably will not last, but how long does that shower you took this morning last? Maybe a day? Does that mean it was a waste of time? It is true that to stay motivated you need do positive things on a daily basis. Otherwise, the mind begins to smell bad just like your body would if you did not shower. Reading positive material, especially in your area of interest, is helpful. Listening to positive and inspiring CDs and watching educational videos is worthwhile.

It all starts with the decision to have the right attitude and choose how you want to see yourself. Positive visualization will help you manifest your goals into reality.

An optimistic attitude is a good predictor of the outcome you want. This goes beyond just putting on a positive face. True optimism is a belief that you can and will hit your target. It is a belief that setbacks are only temporary and there is always something good about that setback. Perhaps just learning what does not work is the most valuable lesson. Sometimes the setback actually will lead to something even better, or put you in touch with a valuable contact.

Optimists believe there is a massive conspiracy to help them succeed. Everything that happens is for their benefit. Pessimists, on the other hand, believe the opposite. The universe and the odds are overwhelmingly stacked against them. This attitude can justify not beginning at all or giving up. In Dr. Seligman's great book, *Learned Optimism,* he talks about optimism being the number one predictor of success.

Basically, optimistic people share these traits. Optimists will:

- Think about what they want and how to get it. They avoid thinking about what they do not want.
- Look for the good in everything, including adversity.
- Seek the valuable lesson in every problem and recover from problems quickly.
- Feed their minds positive material.
- Have visions that stretch them. They will be unrealistic because realistic usually means lowering the bar.
- Try more things. Success is a numbers game. Trying more things means you put the odds in your favor.
- Persist longer. Failure is viewed as temporary and not a reason to stop.

Remember, attitude is a choice. Choose optimism.

2. Use language as a tool to help you. Talk like you are guaranteed success. It is only logical that if you say you want something, like to lose twenty pounds for example, and continually say things like, *"I can never lose weight,"* or, *"My parents were heavy so there's nothing I can do about it,"* you are sabotaging yourself because you do not have a conviction that you can do it. You are creating a plan for failure with the excuses already in place.

Language your way to improvement. Only talk in positives. Don't blame and don't complain. Your body believes every word you say. Instead, change your physiology and your life by your beliefs and your words. Affirmations are a great way to actually program your brain and nervous system for goal achievement. Writing positive statements about what you want to achieve daily will do wonders. When you do affirmations you are literally building new neuronal pathways in your brain that will enable you to think differently. That is how powerful they are.

Three simple rules will help make your affirmations more effective:

A. Begin an affirmation with a positive statement like *I am* or *I have*. Replace all negative words in your affirmations like *don't* or *can't*. For example, "*I am exercising four days a week for forty-five minutes each session.*"

B. Include a time frame in your affirmation. For example, "*I have lost ten pounds by March 15, 2011.*" What if you do not make that target date? That's simple, just revise the date. Some people balk at this exercise because the statement is not true now. What you are doing is programming yourself to make it true.

C. Write them in ink, so the universe knows you're serious.

As you increasingly believe it, you will act as if it were true until it is a reality. Affirmations are a way to create congruency with your goals and beliefs. The idea is to surround yourself with as much positive input as possible so it propels you in the direction you want to wind up.

Some sample affirmations are:

"I have a 32-inch waist by August 15, 2011."
"I love to exercise."
"Every day in every way I am better and better."
"I have completed a mini marathon by January 15, 2012."
"I am a goal-oriented person."
"I only do what gets me closer to my goals."

"I have abundant energy to accomplish all my
  goals."
"I am learning new and valuable things every day."
"I attract all the right people to help me on my
  path."

3. Take action every day. Make a plan of action and break it down into daily steps. Nothing happens until you take action. As the saying goes, *when you meditate, move your feet.* Chopping your goal into bite-sized pieces is helpful. Sometimes it is necessary to keep chopping for awhile. Keep the pieces small enough so you are inspired to do them. As you finish the pieces, the puzzle will come together, and eventually become clear. Momentum will build and your enthusiasm will increase. Instead of it feeling like a chore to do, you will eagerly want to get back to the action steps at every available opportunity.

Prioritizing the steps is necessary to reach your goals. Determine what one thing will make the biggest difference and benefit everything else you do? What is the next important? Then focus on doing something daily.

When you focus on one step each day, goals do not seem so enormous. Focusing also helps build your momentum as you accumulate these daily successes with the prioritized pieces of your goal. When Universal Laws are discussed, the Law of Action is missing much of the time. Do not make that mistake because again *nothing happens until you take action.*

4. Have a good support team. This is essential. You do not have to do it alone and you shouldn't try. A good team on your side can make the difference between succeeding or not. When the great basketball player Michael Jordan first came into professional basketball he scored points like crazy. He racked up amazing personal statistics, but his team never won a championship. It was only when the team added a new coach and different players, and they started working together, that they began to complement each other's strengths as a team and the championships started to come. Jordan was the first to proclaim, "*Nobody does it alone.*"

You should have personal support teams and professional support teams. On a personal level, you should surround yourself with cheerleaders. Be around people who believe in and encourage you. The critics and others who love to pour cold water on your dreams have to go. They are too expensive to associate with on a regular basis. Make no mistake about it: They do have an influence on you.

I realize it can be difficult to separate yourself from all negative people, especially if you are living with one of these people or are related to one. As far as your relatives are concerned, if they persist in their negativity, then you must limit your contact to holidays only, for example. If you are living with a spouse who does not support and cheer you on, something must change. As the great speaker, Les Brown, puts it, *"You can't fight in the arena of life and go home and fight there, too."* You want somebody in your corner that believes in and encourages you, somebody who revives you and gives you the feeling that everything is going to be just fine no matter what.

On a professional level, surrounding yourself with helpful people makes all the difference in the world. Having others do tasks that you do not like to do is a good place to start. Chances are that you are not really good at what you do not like to do anyway. When you are doing that task, it also pulls you away from what you are good at and should be spending most of your time doing. For example, I do not like detail work. I mean, I really do not like it. So I hire someone else to do it. That is so liberating because it takes those jobs off my plate and allows me to only do what I enjoy.

A good support team, to me, is the personnel I hire to help me in the office and at home. These include a sharp bookkeeper and CPA, an educated mechanic, dentist, chiropractors and other doctors, a wise therapist, and other experts in their fields whom I can call with questions, like coaches and mentors. You may want to utilize a personal trainer if you want to expedite your exercise program, for example. If you are having difficulty with, *"How am I going to do this"* kinds of questions, a life coach may be your answer.

As I heard Robert Kyosaki, author of *Rich Dad, Poor Dad,* say, *"I am not very bright, but I surround myself with very bright people."* He obviously is very bright but the point of having a team to give you expert input is so valuable. You can't be an expert in every area. He also does not allow anyone to tell him something can't be done. His philosophy is there is always a way. The task is to find it. When I realized that people at the top did not start there and had help to get where they are, I realized I should do the same thing.

I used to think I had to do it all alone. To be honest, I never got where I wanted to be by doing everything myself. I am now a big believer in using coaches. Coaches can help you cut through the fog and bring clarity to a situation. There are life coaches, business coaches, and coaches that specialize in specific areas, like public speaking. Most people who have achieved superior results have used coaches. In fact, most good coaches even use coaches.

Along with providing good advice, a coach also keeps you accountable. Sometimes it can be challenging to do the necessary action steps. With a coach on your side advising, supporting, and encouraging you, the impossible becomes possible. Writing this book is a perfect example. It remained a wish for over twenty years. It wasn't until I incorporated the help of an excellent support team to cheer me on the path of completing my goal that I was inspired to finish it. You will have the confidence it will happen, it is just a matter of time. With a coach keeping you on track with your commitments, before you know it, your goal will be a reality. Remember Michael Jordan's words, "*Nobody does it alone.*" My advice is do not try. It is the hard way and you'll waste too much time.

5. Choose not to stress. Stress is an obstacle that will age you faster, cause disease, and can even kill you. The experience of excessive stress is really where every disease begins. There is not one good thing about stress unless you need to run away from a tiger or dodge arrows. In other words, if you are unexpectedly facing a life-threatening situation, you would want to experience the physiological and physical changes of the stress response, but to live like you are trying to save your life all the time is a killer. So many people are ready to burst and any little thing will make them explode.

A good form of self therapy is when you are feeling stressed, take action over something you can control, like cleaning out your closets. Anthony Robbins says to look at any stressful or negatively-perceived event and ask first what you can learn from it and then what the opportunity is. There is always an answer to these two questions. Your challenge is to stay calm and clear enough to ask the questions and see the answers. This is why many times a seemingly negative event will turn out to be a very good thing. People will often say things like, *"That's the best thing that ever happened to me"* later on.

It is important to recharge our batteries as an antidote to stress. Find what brings you a feeling of peace and calm. For me, watching ocean waves roll onto the sand or being near a high mountain stream definitely does it. The mind can only consciously think of one thing at a time. Surround yourself with favorite pictures or objects that make you think of positive memories. I have pictures of nature scenes in my office that bring me peace. I also play music that is pleasant and soothing.

If a stressful situation arises, just focus on the positive picture or object and it can immediately start to alleviate the feelings of stress. Will it eliminate the stressor? Probably not, but remember when we are feeling stress our brains are not functioning as sharply. This technique will give us a break and help focus more clearly. Remember that stress can only affect you if you let it in. All the water in the ocean can't sink a ship unless it gets inside. By focusing on the positive you are not letting stress get inside you. To let stress in is just too big of a price to pay.

6. Always have an eraser handy. To be results oriented, it is necessary to make adjustments from time to time. Sometimes, if we are honest with ourselves, we will see that something is not working. How do we know it is not working? The results we are getting (or not getting) are our way of measuring the effectiveness of our plan. The point is, if the results are not there, we should be ready and willing to erase our old way of doing things and be open to try something new or different.

If your goal was to lose ten pounds in three months and you gained five pounds instead, obviously your action plan did not work. *You need to examine your plan, tweak , or throw it out all together and start over.* I have noticed high achievers do this because they are so focused on getting results. Most high level athletes are like this as well. The majority of people however, do just the opposite. Even though what they are doing does not work, they will keep on doing it, defend it, and argue with those who point out that what they are doing does not work. For whatever reason, they have their ego invested in it, or they have a resistance to other ideas, or what they are doing goes along with an erroneous belief they have.

It has nothing to do with intelligence, but most people will only let into their brains what fits their current belief systems. The results oriented person is open to examining those beliefs and is willing to erase them as well and replace them with new beliefs that will lead to progress, not stagnation.

It is an amazing phenomenon to observe someone defending something that obviously does not work, yet watch how often people do it. There are many deep issues that can interfere with clear thinking. I know a consultant who receives a high fee for his services and all he does is go into someone's office and observe what is not working and change it immediately. If there is an employee that hasn't worked out for example, the consultant will rectify the situation that day. Usually the owner of the business has known for some time the employee is not a good fit, yet does not know how to fix it, has a fear of confrontation, or perhaps another reason.

The point is to be truly effective there has to be zero tolerance for what does not work. Nothing positive will result from continuing to go along with things that are sabotaging your progress.

Fix, eliminate, or replace, and the sooner the better. Continue to focus on your results and what it takes to get there. Do not worry about who gets credit for what or what the neighbors think. Chances are they are not thinking about you anyway. Be willing to erase as often as necessary and make changes until you reach your destination.

CONCLUSION

Thank you for your interest in *Turn Back the Clock*. My sincerest wish is that you got something from these pages that will make a big difference for you. Please keep in mind that knowledge without action will not produce results. My recommendation is to start with baby steps in a particular area of needed improvement. Inch by inch, life is a cinch. The important thing is to do a little each day.

I welcome your experiences utilizing the principles in this book. You may call me at (916) 962-3101 or my email address is: dcrawforddc@sbcglobal.net. Good luck!

INDEX

A

acacia, 118, 131

acetaminophen, 112

N-acetyl cysteine (NAC), 30, 31, 48, 138

acetyl L-carnitine, 36

acetylcholine, 27, 33, 36

addiction, chronic worry as, 71, 74–75

adrenal glands, 57–58, 71, 135
    stress and, 71, 120, 125
    support for, 119

affirmations, 178–180

alfalfa, 124, 129

aloe, 118

aluminum, 30

Alzheimer's disease, 27, 36

American ginseng, 58, 124, 126, 128

amylase, 113, 157

anthocyanins, 32

antiaging support, 134–140

antibiotics, 100–102, 152
    natural, 116–118

antigliadin antibody test, 30

antioxidants, 29, 115, 134–135, 139
    coenzyme Q10 as, 54
    depletion of, 27

antivirals, natural, 118

Applied Kinesiology, 121–122

artemesia annua, 123, 130

ashwagandha, 58, 119

aspirin, 90, 112, 114
    side effects of regular use, 91–92
astaxanthin, 134–135
astragalus, 118, 128
ATP (adenosine triphosphate), 31, 53, 133
attention deficit disorder, 27
avocados, 145

B

B vitamins, 36. See also specific vitamins
back pain, 55
    intestinal connection to, 122–123, 149–150
    kidney stress and, 123–125
    nervous system imbalance and, 125–127
bananas, 124, 134
barberry, 118
beet juice, 132, 133
berberine, 111, 123, 130
berries, 32
bile, 151
black cohosh, 136
black walnuts, 123
blood sugar
    high blood pressure and, 94
    imbalance in, 22
    natural remedies to normalize, 120–121
blueberries, 32, 132
boneset, 117, 140
boron, 140
brain
    activities benefiting, 37–38

foods promoting health of, 32–33

glucose availability to, 22

inflammation in, 26

oxygen supply to, 21

stress hormones and, 68

support for, 35–37

bromelain, 113

C

calcium d-glucarate, 31, 48

calcium hydroxyapatite, 140

cancer, 29, 144, 146, 157

antioxidants and, 115

breast, 46, 136

colon, 35, 93

folic acid and, 52

magnesium and, 51

pancreatic, aspirin and, 92

carbohydrates

complex, 145–146

digestion of, 157

refined, 50, 120, 145

cardiovascular disease, natural remedies for, 132–134

Carel, Alexis, 65

Carnegie, Dale, 80

L-carnitine, 54, 132

L-carnosine, 37

cascara sagrada, 130

celery/celery juice, 113–114, 132, 134

chi gong, 24

chia seeds, 139, 145

chlorella, 31, 138–139
chlorophyll, 120, 138
cholesterol, 54–55, 151
    eggs and, 144
    myths about, 86–90
choline, 33
cilantro, 31
cissus quadrangularis, 140
coenzyme Q10, 35–37, 54–55, 89, 132
coffee, 148–149
colds/flu. see also flu vaccines/vaccination
    remedies for, 115, 116, 128
collagen, 136–137
colostrum, 153
congestive heart failure, 89
constipation, natural remedies for, 130–131
cortisol, 57, 71, 136
cranberry, 117
C-reactive protein (CRP), 29

D

deglycyrrhizinated licorice (DGL), 111
dehydration, 33, 147, 148
DeMartini, John, 59
DHA, 36
DHEA (dehydroepiendosterone), 135–136
diet(s), 141–149. See also food
    cholesterol in, 87
    high-sugar, 50, 134
    low-cholesterol, 89–90
    standard American, 142

digestion
    importance of enzymes in, 161
    process of, 150–151
digestive problems. See also gastrointestinal problems
    causes of, 152–153, 154
    dysbiosis, 51, 130–131
    musculoskeletal problems and, 149–150
D-mannose, 117
dopamine, 27
dysbiosis, 51, 130–131

E

ear infections, 101–102
echinacea, 117
eggs, 33, 144
emotions, toxic, 48–49
energy
    ATP and, 31, 53
    depleted, factors influencing, 41–42
    exercise and, 22–23, 38
    important nutrients for, 50
    muscle, 89, 132–133
    spleen and, 43
    stress and, 55–56, 67–68
    supplements boosting, 136, 137, 138–139
enzyme therapists, 45
enzymes
    anti-inflammatory, 113
    aspirin and, 92
    circumstances depleting/destroying, 159–161
    digestive, 45, 120, 150–151

importance of, 154–159
proteolytic, 123, 124, 140
essential fatty acids (EFAs), 50, 54, 113, 132
role of, 53
eucalyptus, 118
excitotoxins, 35
exercise, 22
for back pain, 127–128
benefits to brain, 38
in eleviation of worry/stress, 69
overexertion in, 23–24

F

fatigue, 26, 41
fat(s)
hydrogenated, 26, 34, 54
natural, 145
utilization of, 23–24
fatty acids, 44, 50, 113. See also essential fatty acids
DHA, 36
omega-3, 32
Feldenkrais Method®, 70
fennel, 130
fight or flight response, 67
flax, 145
flu, remedies for, 115, 116, 128
flu vaccines/vaccination, 30–31, 47–48
fluoride, 31, 35
folic acid (vitamin B9), 29, 50, 52, 88
food irradiation, 160, 167–168
foods. See also processed foods

to avoid, 33–35
marketed as healthy, 96–98
promoting brain health, 32–33
triggering gall bladder discomfort, 151
fractures, natural remedies promoting healing of, 140
free radicals, 26–27, 88
activity in fatty tissue, marker for, 28
dementia and, 116
stress and production of, 39

G

GABA, 119
gall bladder, 151–152
gall stones, 151
garlic, 116, 123, 130
gastrointestinal problems
antibiotics and, 102
from aspirin use, 91
back pain and, 122–123, 149–150
dysbiosis, 51, 130–131
garlic and, 116
ileocecal valve problems, 119–120
natural remedies for, 110–112
stress and, 68
gentleness, 37
ginger, 114–115, 116
ginseng, 58, 124, 126, 128
glucuronidation detox pathway, 31–32, 48
glutathione, 29–30, 36, 53, 138
acetaminophen and, 112, 115
synthesis of, 138

gluten intolerance, test for, 30
goals
    avoiding stress over, 184–186
    barriers to achieving, 165–175
    having right attitude/optimism about, 175–178
    language/affirmations as tools for, 178–180
    revising, 186–188
    setting, 61, 163–164
    support teams and, 181–184
    taking daily action toward, 180–181
goldenseal, 116–117, 131
grape juice, 133
grape seed extract, 36
grapefruit seed extract, 111, 117, 123, 130, 131
gymnema sylvestre, 120

H

happiness, steps to promote, 80–83
hawthorne, 133
headache, 115
    major causes of, 118–121
heartburn, 92
high blood pressure (HBP), 93–95
    aspirin and, 91
    natural remedies for, 131–132
high fructose corn syrup, 146–147
homocysteine, 28–29, 88
How to Stop Worrying and Start Living (Carnegie), 80
hydrogenated fats, 26, 34, 54
5 hydroxytryptophan (5-HTP), 119

I

ileocecal valve (ICV) problems, 119–120
iliacus muscle, 120, 122
immune system
    antibiotics and, 102
    fatigue and, 42–43
    natural boosters of, 128–129
indigestion, 92–93
infection(s)
    natural antibiotics for, 116–118
    undiagnosed, fatigue and, 41–42
inflammation
    fatigue and, 44
    natural remedies for, 112–116
    screening tests for, 28–30
insecticides, 31, 160
intestinal problems. See gastrointestinal problems
isatis, 118

J

joints/joint pain, 43
    bromelain and, 113
    collagen supplementation for, 137
    ginger and, 115
    sacroiliac (SI), 125–127
    vitamin K and, 129
juniper, 117

K

kidneys
    aspirin use and, 91
    back pain and, 123–125
    stresses on, 93, 94, 112, 136
    support for, 33, 37, 51, 129

L

leaky gut syndrome, 42–43
learning, 37
lecithin, 33, 144
Leon, Keith, 61
licorice, 58, 128, 134
    deglycyrrhizinated (DGL), 111
lifestyle habits, benefiting brain, 38–39
lipase, 113, 145, 158
lipid peroxidation, 26, 28, 35
lipoid acid, 30, 36, 50, 138
    benefits of, 31, 37, 53
liver, 35, 52, 54
    acetaminophen and, 112
    aspirin and, 91
    detoxification systems of, 31–32
    migraines and, 121
    statin use and, 89
    stress and, 66
    support for, 48, 53
    turmeric and, 115

M

maca, 139
magnesium, 31, 50–51, 88
   cardiovascular heath and, 133–134
   migraines and, 121
maitake mushroom, 128
manganese, 140
Maximum Achievement (Tracy), 71–72
meals, timing of, 147
meats, processed, 34–35, 143–144
meditation, 69, 70, 94, 136
mercury, 30, 31
methionine, 28, 88
methylation cycle, 28
microwave cooking, 160–161
   lipid peroxidation and, 26
milk
   mother's, 152–153
   pasteurization of, 160
   raw, 153–154
mitochondria, 22, 26, 132
movement with focus/slow movement exercise, 24, 37
MSG (monosodium glutamate), 35, 143
mullein, 124
muscle(s)/muscle pain
   bromelain and, 113
   coenzyme Q10 and, 54, 89, 132
   collagen supplementation and, 137
   digestive issues and, 149–150
   exercise and, 24
   gluteus maximus, 126

iliacus, 120, 122
magnesium and, 24
quadratus lumborum, 123–124
Sartorius, 125

N

nattokinase, 133
natural medicine paradigm, 106
natural remedies, 108
    antibiotic, 116–118
    antiviral, 118
    for blood sugar imbalance, 120–121
    for cardiovascular disease, 132–134
    exceptions to use of, 109
    for high blood pressure, 131–132
    for inflammation, 112–116
    for pain, 112–116
    for stomach pain, 110–112
nettles, 136
Neuro Emotional Technique (NET), 70
neurotransmitters, 27
    stress and production of, 39
non-steroidal anti-inflammatory drugs, 112
NutraSweet TM, 35
nutrient depletion, fatigue and, 51–55

O

oils
    with anti-inflammatory action, 113
    rancid, 26, 35

omega-3 fatty acids, 32
optimism/optimists, 176–178
oregano, 123
Oregon grape root, 118
oxidative stress test, 28

P

pain, natural remedies for, 112–116
pancreas, 155–156
pantothenic acid. See vitamin B5
Parkinson's disease, 27, 36
parsley, 124, 129
pasta, 146
phosphatidylserine, 36
potassium, 51, 133, 134
Pottinger's Saucer, 149
pregnenolone, 135, 136
prescription drugs, 46–47
    antioxidant depletion and, 27
    myths about, 98–100
    potassium-depleting, 134
    psychotropic, 28
probiotics, 120, 123, 130, 131
processed foods, 34–35, 52, 142–143
    enzyme deficiencies and, 158–159
prostaglandins, 91
prostate support, 136
protease deficiency, 156–157
proteins
    increased water intake with, 147
    sources of, 145

undigested, 93
   whey, 30, 138
psychotropic drugs, 28
pumpkin seed, 136
purposeful living, 58–61
pygeum, 136
pyridoxal-5'–phosphate (P5P), 52

Q

Quantum Neurology®, 102

R

red clover, 136
red wine, 121, 135
reishi mushroom, 128–129
relationships, toxic, 49–50
responsibility, accepting, 168–169
resveratrol, 36, 135
Rhodiola, 58
riboflavin, 30, 121, 138
D-ribose, 133

S

sacroiliac (SI) joint, 125–127
sage, 117
salmon, wild, 32, 53
saw palmetto, 136
selenium, 30, 31, 44, 48, 138
self-examination, 20

senna, 130
serotonin, 27, 88–89, 159
Shiitake mushroom, 128
Shillings Test, 52
Siberian ginseng, 58, 128
silver fillings, 30
sinus infections, 100–101
SIRT1 gene, 36
sleep, 38–39, 55, 130
sodium, 114
soft drinks, 146–147
soy, 145
spinach, 33
spirulina, 138
spleen, 43, 128, 152
statins, 54, 132
    side effects of, 89
stress
    control of, 39, 68–70, 184–186
    fatigue and, 55–58
    worry and, 66–68
sugar(s)
    artificial, 147
    refined, 98, 142–143, 146
support teams, 181–183

T

tai chi, 24
Tarahamara Indians, 139
thiamin. See vitamin B1
thymus, 43, 128

thyroid
    cholesterol and, 87–88
    imbalance in, fatigue and, 44
tongkat ali, 136
toxicity, fatigue and, 45–50
toxins
    avoidance of, 30–31
    liver detoxification of, 31–32
    neurological, 26–27
    sources of, 45–48
Tracy, Brian, 71–72
tribulus, 136
turmeric, 114, 115–116, 138

U

upper limit problem, 71–75
usnea, 117
uva ursi, 117

V

vaccines/vaccinations, 30–31
    myths about, 95–96
velvet deer antler, 136
vitamin A, 129
vitamin B1 (thiamin), 51, 132–133
vitamin B5 (pantothenic acid), 58
vitamin B6, 52, 88
vitamin B9. See folic acid
vitamin B12, 52–53, 88
vitamin C, 129, 135, 144

vitamin K2, 140

W

Walker, Scott, 70
walnuts, 32, 145
    black, 123
water, 33, 148
    increasing, with increased protein intake, 147
wellness, associated with brain health, 19–20
wheat germ oil, 113
wheat grass, 138
wheat/wheat flour, 146, 151, 152, 154
whey proteins, 30, 138, 145
Who Do You think You Are (Leon), 61
Why Zebras Don't Get Ulcers (Solposki), 67
wine, red, 121, 135
worry
    as cause of stress, 55–56
    common sources of, 64–65
    as learned behavior, 70–71
    physiological/physical effects of, 66–67
    steps to eliminate, 75–80
    upper limit problem and, 71–75

Y

yeast, 123, 130, 159
    natural antibiotics against, 116, 117
yoga, 24, 121–122
yucca, 113

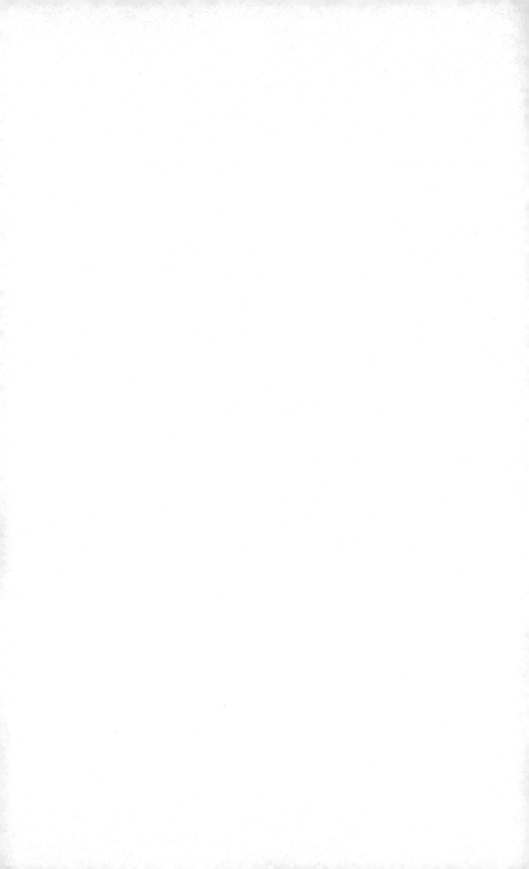

*Question: I loved Dr. Crawford's book,
how can I continue to work with him?*

*Answer: Dr. Crawford has created a DVD Video Series
on many of the subjects covered in this book. These
"Live" presentations are full of valuable
and life altering information.*

Take advantage of these Introductory Specials right now at:

www.CrawfordNaturalHealthCenter.com/dvds-products

NATURAL REMEDIES FOR COMMON AILMENTS

- Why natural is better

- Natural immune boosters

- What to do for colds and viruses

- Treating coughs naturally

- Dealing with injuries, pain, and inflammation

- Natural antibiotics

CANCER-TREATMENTS AND PREVENTION

- What exactly is cancer?

- The cancer epidemic nobody talks about

- What are some of the causes?

- Treatments and options

- Foods for prevention

- And more

HEALTH MYTHS

- Is an aspirin a day really healthy?
- Is low cholesterol really healthy?
- Why your appendix is NOT worthless
- Indigestion is not caused by excess acid
- Are vaccination and immunization the same?
- High blood pressure is not a disease

TRICK OR TREATMENT

- Muscle testing as a therapeutic tool
- Applying the Law of 5 Elements
- Tricks to be aware of
- The healing power of cold laser light
- Why people move themselves into dysfunction
- Color, sound, and smell as healing aids

SACRED MEDICINE-ANCIENT WISDOM

- Plants as medicine
- Animals as teachers
- Using feathers and journey staffs
- The four sacred paths
- Ceremony and plants

FOODS, MOODS, AND BEHAVIOR

- The brain and behavior
- Why the Standard American Diet is SAD

- What we can learn from athletes
- The diet-behavior connection
- How neurotoxins are destroying us
- Foods for mood control

HEALTHY AGING

- Maintain strong bones
- Keep your immune system robust
- Sharpen your memory
- Increase flexibility
- Improve balance

ENJOY SPRING: FREE FROM ALLERGIES, HEADACHES & CONGESTION – Learn natural and healthy remedies to prevent:

- Itchy, irritated eyes
- Stuffy, runny nose
- Sinus headaches, congestion and more

AVOIDING STRESS IN STRESSFUL SITUATIONS (Like the Holidays)

- Learn to manage stress more effectively
- Stabilize your moods: the "food-mood" connection
- Supplements to keep you sane and that keep your energy up
- Simple de-stress techniques, and how to deal with "difficult" people and more

THE PATH TO DIABETES

- Learn how not to become a statistic

- Warning signs of impending trouble and the seriousness of diabetes

- The REAL causes of diabetes and the role stress plays

- Diet and supplements to control, and even reverse, type 2 diabetes, and more

LIFE IS BETTER WITH BALANCED HORMONES – (For Men and Women) Learn what you can do for life to go more smoothly, for you and yours

- Herbs, supplements and foods for hormone balance

- Alleviating PMS symptoms and sailing through menopause

- Why infertility is epidemic, how to prevent prostate and breast problems and more

HEART HEALTH NATURALLY – Learn the truth about heart disease

- What lab tests should be done to spot impending danger

- The real problem regarding cholesterol (you'll be surprised)

- Is aspirin a health food? Blocked arteries – causes and cures

- Foods and nutrients that support your cardiovascular system

- The role of exercise and emotions

- Why high blood pressure is not a disease

TREATING ARTHRITIS AND JOINT PAIN – Learn what it is and how to prevent it

- Where does arthritis come from? Warning signs of trouble ahead

- How to control the pain and inflammation

- Regenerating damaged joints, The best exercises and diet

- Nutrients to resolve arthritis symptoms

HEREDITY, HABITS AND HEALTH – Learn to create your own future

- Are we really victims of our heredity? How genes are affected by beliefs

- The most important factors affecting our health: steps for positive change

- Understanding natural laws and how to work with them

MESSAGES FROM THE HEART – Why our heart intelligence is the main factor in our lives

- The heart-brain connection

- The damaging effects of stress

- How to transform stress

- Increase your energy using heart intelligence

- The heart and emotional maturity

- Tools to change your life now

STOP WORRYING – START LIVING

- What is worry and where does it come from?

- Why the subconscious mind will automatically trigger worry

- The effects of worry on our health

- Action steps to eliminate worry

- The way to peace and happiness

INTESTINAL INTELLIGENCE

- How the abdomen operates as a "second brain"

- Why nerve messengers made in the gut are as important as ones made in the brain

- How most of the body's immune system is in the abdomen

- "Gut Instincts" – How the gut is always talking to you

- Why the brain and the "abdominal brain" must be in sync, and what happens when they are not

- Simple techniques for intestinal health that will slow the aging process

FEELING FINE IN 2009 – Making resolutions a reality

- Staying focused, making changes, purpose and passion

- Make health a priority resolution, living conscientiously

BEGIN AGAIN IN 2010

- Why making New Year's resolutions rarely works

- Keeping our focus on improvement

- Why optimism is essential and learnable

- How to get in shape mentally and physically

- Power of purpose and congruency

- 7 tips for a great year

"I have truly enjoyed Dr. Crawford's lectures. Dr. Crawford delivers his messages professionally and with a sense of humor. I have gotten rid of many day-to-day pressures by implementing several of Dr. Crawford's practical suggestions into my daily life."
– M. Carotti

Order you DVD copies right now at:
www.CrawfordNaturalHealthCenter.com/dvds-products

To receive Dr. Dennis K. Crawford's Newsletter go to:
www.CrawfordNaturalHealthCenter.com

For a phone consultation with Dr. Crawford,
call (916) 962-3101

Email Dr. Crawford for a complimentary DVD
titled: Beyond Food

Topics Include:
1. Six basic rules for healthy eating that will change your life
2. Why a quality diet is only part of the answer
3. Why the Standard American Diet (SAD) can only bring about sad results
4. Why diets don't usually work
5. Why we all need help with digestion
6. The importance of enzymes to health
7. And more...

Made in the USA
Monee, IL
24 February 2021